Collaborative Learning in Practice

Coaching to Support Student Learners in Healthcare

Charlene Lobo, BSc, MA, RN, RHV
Independent Consultant Practice Education
UK

Rachel Paul, BA, MA
Director
ConsultEast
Norwich, England, UK

Kenda Crozier, PhD, MSc, BSc, RM, RN, SFHEA
Professor of Midwifery
Director for International Partnerships
School of Health Sciences
Faculty of Medicine and Health Sciences
University of East Anglia
Norwich, England, UK

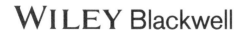

WILEY Blackwell

This edition first published 2021
© 2021 John Wiley & Sons Ltd.

The right of Charlene Lobo, Rachel Paul, and Kenda Crozier to be identified as the authors of this work has been asserted in accordance with law.

Registered Offices
John Wiley & Sons, Inc., 111 River Street, Hoboken, NJ 07030, USA
John Wiley & Sons Ltd, The Atrium, Southern Gate, Chichester, West Sussex, PO19 8SQ, UK

Editorial Office
9600 Garsington Road, Oxford, OX4 2DQ, UK

For details of our global editorial offices, customer services, and more information about Wiley products visit us at www.wiley.com.

Wiley also publishes its books in a variety of electronic formats and by print-on-demand. Some content that appears in standard print versions of this book may not be available in other formats.

Library of Congress Cataloging-in-Publication Data

Names: Lobo, Charlene, 1957- author. | Paul, Rachel, 1960- author. |
    Crozier, Kenda, 1963- author.
Title: Collaborative learning in practice : coaching to support student
    learners in healthcare / Charlene Lobo, Rachel Paul, Kenda Crozier.
Description: First edition. | Hoboken, NJ : Wiley-Blackwell, 2021. |
    Includes bibliographical references and index.
Identifiers: LCCN 2020050275 (print) | LCCN 2020050276 (ebook) | ISBN
    9781119695363 (paperback) | ISBN 9781119695387 (adobe pdf) | ISBN
    9781119695424 (epub)
Subjects: LCSH: Nurses–Training of. | Nursing–Study and teaching. | Group
    work in education. | Nurses–Law and legislation–Great Britain. |
    Midwives–Law and legislation–Great Britain.
Classification: LCC RT71 .L57 2021 (print) | LCC RT71 (ebook) | DDC
    610.73076–dc23
LC record available at https://lccn.loc.gov/2020050275
LC ebook record available at https://lccn.loc.gov/2020050276

Cover Design: Wiley
Cover Image: © sturti/E+/Getty Images

Set in 9.5/12.5pt STIXTwoText by Straive, Chennai, India
Printed and bound by CPI Group (UK) Ltd, Croydon, CR0 4YY

C9781119695363_100521

Collaborative Learning in Practice

This book is dedicated to all mentors, supervisors, practice educators, and coaches supporting the future workforce. We hope this book will make practice learning a really positive experience and inspire you to be even more powerful practice educators. Students past and present owe you a debt of gratitude which they can pay forward to the next generation.

Contents

Collaborator Biographies

Tony Arthur
Tony Arthur is Professor of Nursing Science at the University of East Anglia. He is also a nurse at the Norfolk and Norwich University Hospitals Foundation NHS Trust where he works on an acute older people's medical ward. He has led and collaborated on a range of research studies, where his interests lie in the evaluation of nursing interventions for older people and the epidemiology of ageing. He has degrees in Sociology, Medical Statistics, and Epidemiology.

Dr Helen Bell, PhD, MSc, PGCEA, RNT, BSc (Hons), RN, PMRAFNS
Dr Helen Bell is an Associate Professor in Adult Nursing, Practice Education Lead for Adult Nursing, and Academic Lead for Equality, Diversity, and Inclusion at University of East Anglia. She has been involved in nurse education for 27 years, specialisng in aeromedical nursing in the RAF and critical care nursing. She supports a diverse range of learners in clinical practice including direct entry nursing students, accelerated pre-registration master's students, and nursing degree/nursing associate apprentices, their practice supervisors/assessors, and clinical educators, across a broad spectrum of regional healthcare placements, many of whom have adopted the CLiP™ model or adaptations thereof. Her research interests focus on the factors that contribute to success in pre-registration nurse education.

Jane Bunce
Jane Bunce has worked in medical education since 2005 and currently works for Health Education England (HEE) as Quality Lead in the South

West. Jane's own educational achievements include a First Class Degree in Business Studies and an MSc in Healthcare Leadership. Following her Masters, Jane undertook a HEE Fellowship to extend her interest in research and this led to her collaboration with the University of Plymouth on several research projects related to the development of Collaborative Learning in Practice in the South West. Jane successfully project managed the HEE SW CLiP Community Cluster Project in 2018/2019, which piloted the approach in GP, care home, and hospice settings. Most recently, she is leading the HEE CLiP PCN project in the South West which aims to explore how the benefits of the model across primary care networks.

Professor Kenda Crozier, PhD, MSc, PGDip, BSc, RM, RN
Kenda Crozier is Professor of Midwifery at the University of East Anglia. She has been involved in nursing and midwifery education for 20 years, with experience in developing curricula in nursing and midwifery that include interprofessional practice, enquiry based learning at undergraduate level, advanced practice programmes for health professions at Masters level, and postgraduate research training programmes for doctoral students. Her interest in CLiP began with a University of East Anglia visit to VU Amsterdam where she experienced it in action. Recently, she has run workshops with Health Education England to promote collaborative learning in practice for midwifery education. Her current educational research is exploring the current development of advanced practice in midwifery.

Rebekah Hill
Rebekah Hill works as an Associate Professor within the School of Health Sciences, University of East Anglia. Her role involves teaching and assessing both undergraduate and postgraduate healthcare practitioners across a range of professions. Rebekah now works as the Director of Education in the school and has a special interest in assessment of learning. Rebekah works clinically as an advanced life support instructor and within gastroenterology nursing, maintaining her special interest in hepatitis C.

Mr David Huggins
Senior Lecturer/Course Director Operating Department Practice

After training in the National Health Service (NHS) in 1984 as an operating department assistant (ODA) at the James Paget University Hospital in Gorleston on Sea, Norfolk, I worked in many other areas including London, Manchester, and Norwich as well as a period overseas as a cardiac technician in St Vincent's Hospital Sydney, New South Wales.

I became training lead for ODAs in Harrogate in the early 1990s and gained various teaching and assessing qualification during this time. In 1995, I moved to the Norfolk and Norwich University Hospital where I was employed as a Senior Operating Department Practitioner (SODP) and was responsible for not only training of ODPs but staff development too. In 2003, ODP training entered Higher Education (HE) and I was the first lecturer in operating department practice at the University of East Anglia.

As course director, I am actively involved with promoting the operating department practitioner (ODP) role and influencing practice. I have over 30 years' experience of working in a variety of operating theatre settings locally, nationally, and internationally and have a keen interest in all educational matters, especially the vital role that educators and coaches play in supporting and developing learners. I also enjoy delivering post-reg modules and am leadership pathway lead in the School of Health Sciences.

Adele Kane, MSc Health and Social Care Education, RN, RNT, HEA Fellow

Adele Kane is an Associate Head of School Practice Learning with Plymouth University, Programme Lead and Subject Specialist for Return to Practice & Health Education England Peninsular SW Fellow Practice Learning.

She has been programme Lead and Subject Specialist in Mentorship and lead projects in E-Learning development. Through her role with the University and Health Education England she has actively supported the implementation of Collaborative Learning in Practice (CliP) Projects within the majority of Acute and Community Hospital care settings for Adult, Mental Health and Midwifery students in the southwest. More recently, leading a project within the private sector with GP Practices, Hospices and Care Homes. Currently a consultant advisor for Health Education England in a joint project with Southwest HEI's to introduce CLIP within Primary care networks as a next step forward.

Jonty Kenward

Jonty has been a qualified nurse for 25 years, her clinical background was in community practice, and as an anaesthetic nurse. For the past seven years, she has worked in a number of roles in practice education including, clinical tutor, practice education facilitator (PEF), and CLiP lead where she introduced and developed CLiP within the hospital Trust. Currently, she holds the position of Head of Student Trainee Placement Support, Lancashire Teaching Hospitals NHS Foundation Trust (LTHTR) which involves leading all undergraduate and postgraduate education teams within the organisation. Jonty is passionate about the Collaborative Learning in Practice model for student support and learning; she implemented the CLiP model at LTHTR in 2015, working with her teams to develop this within nursing and midwifery across all acute clinical areas. She has spent the last five years promoting the model nationally and sharing best practice with other higher education institutions and NHS Trusts.

Charlene Lobo, MA Healthcare Education, BSc (Hons.), RN, RHV

Charlene Lobo works as an educational consultant, having spent most of her employed life as a nurse, health visitor, and Senior Lecturer in Public Health and Primary Care at the University of East Anglia. As senior lecturer, she also held the practice education lead in the School of Health Sciences, very much focusing on the quality of the learning environment and how to improve the experiences for both students and mentors. The notion of 'the burden of mentorship' arose from an extensive study over one year collating the feedback from mentors of their experiences of supporting students in practice, and it is from this position that she sought to make a difference and developed the Collaborative Learning in Practice (CLiP™) model of practice learning. This book has brought together her long-time desire to share her insights of the CLiP model from both theoretical and practical perspectives.

Rachel Paul, MA in Professional Development and Education BA (Hons) Business Studies

Rachel worked in the City of London for a pioneering (pre internet) online Information Retrieval company before making a bold decision to leave a secure career and volunteer for VSO in a refugee settlement in Zambia. On her return to the UK Rachel worked helping people to set up co-operative businesses before moving to Lowestoft College delivering business and management training. At Lowestoft College

Rachel undertook her Certificate in Education and then completed a Masters at UEA. In 1999, Rachel moved to the School of Education at Norwich City College, delivering vocational and postgraduate education qualifications. Since 2004, Rachel has run ConsultEast specialising in helping people and teams work better and has built a strong reputation for coaching others in challenging, long-standing and intractable issues. ConsultEast also developed and delivered Institute of Leadership and Management Coaching qualifications at level five and seven. Rachel is qualified as a Cognitive Behaviour Coach and Coaching Supervisor with the Association of Coaching.

Ronald Simpson

Ronnie Simpson was a practice educator for a mental health trust. As part of his role as a Registered Mental Health Nurse he had responsibility for students in the clinical area where CLiP was implemented into Mental Health Practice. He recognised the need and implemented a position to ensure there was a nominated person outside the immediate clinical environment but inside both the education and clinical areas to be an intermediary for learners. He used his experiences to shape and tailor a CLiP programme/package to ensure students experienced a holistic and positive placement.

Kirsty Tweedie

Kirsty is a registered midwife and neonatal examiner with a background as a delivery suite lead both internationally and locally. She has been involved in midwifery education for eight years. She teaches both pre-egistration midwifery and paramedic science and is the lead for the provision of the Neonatal and Infant Physical Examination module which is delivered at MSc level. She had been involved in writing the curricula for the incoming MSci Midwifery programme for which she is the course director. Her interest in CLiP began when she and a practice-based colleague agreed to pilot CLiP as a new way of teaching and learning in practice to bring about a more equitable and student-led learning environment.

Theresa Walker, RN, DN

Theresa Walker worked for nearly 40 years in the NHS as a Registered General Nurse; ten years in an acute hospital setting, twenty years in community nursing and the last decade as a Team Leader in a range of roles, both in inpatient and home care settings. She is completely committed to developing future nurses for working in the community and believes they require a different managerial, organisational and interpersonal skill set than hospital nursing. Theresa feels the community offers great opportunity for novice practitioners and strongly believes that the CLiP model has the ability to give student nurses the opportunity to understand the difference in skill set needed in the community and the opportunity to develop them.

Graham R. Williamson

Dr. Graham R Williamson is an Associate Professor of Adult Nursing at the University of Plymouth School of Nursing and Midwifery, Exeter School of Nursing. He has had a 25-year career in research related to student placement learning and has recently been principal investigator leading a research team investigating CLIP in the South West region, in collaboration with Health Education England. Dr Williamson is currently Editor-in-Chief of the *Open Nursing Journal* (https://opennursingjournal.com). Graham's publications can be accessed via this link https://orcid.org/0000-0002-5715-8621.

Jodie Yerrell, DipHE Midwifery (with Advanced Studies) RM

Jodie Yerrell is a Better Births Lead Midwife, across Norfolk and Waveney Local Maternity and Neonatal System (LMNS), essentially focusing on implementing continuity of carer as a large-scale change. Her other current interests include the Saving Babies' Lives Care Bundle, leading a system-wide safety work stream, and she is a member of the East of England regional work stream. She is currently the LMNS lead for perinatal mental health and is looking forward to the transformation work around maternity and mental health services.

Coaching in midwifery became a real interest for Jodie during her role of midwifery clinical educator at the James Paget University Hospital where she worked closely with University of East Anglia colleagues to successfully lead the implementation of CLiP on the antenatal and postnatal ward. Being the first maternity unit nationally to adopt an alternative to traditional mentorship she was keen to share the success of CLiP and contributed to the planning and delivery of a conference with Health Education England. Jodie also enjoyed working as a practice development midwife in the same Trust.

Jodie is currently a MSc student on the Advanced Midwifery Practice programme at Anglia Ruskin University.

Foreword

There is no greater time to celebrate new learning techniques and bring them to the fore as right now. With the impact of COVID 19 still playing out in our lives, communities, and workplaces we are seeing more innovation, flexibility, and complementary learning opportunities than ever before. From 2020 onwards, we will see the greatest number of generations in the workforce at the same time, greater diversity than seen before, with an increasing mix of skills, experiences, values, and motivations. It is important to understand, cultivate, and make the very best of this opportunity to develop the skills of our workforce now and into the future.

The National People Plan: 'WE ARE THE NHS: People Plan 2020/21 – action for us all' (NHSE/I 2020) launched in July 2020 raises the profile of the importance of learning, support and maximising skills for the workforce right through from apprenticeships, undergraduates, to postgraduate learners, and those wishing to retire who still have an important role to play in supporting skill acquisition in the workforce. It is a relief that this national policy highlights the vital importance of lifelong learning, embraces different approaches, and signposts the increased investment that will be needed to provide the learning and support our workforce needs and deserves.

I have been working in healthcare for 37 years, with 5 years in the independent sector and 32 years in the NHS. If I reflect on my own challenging experiences as a pupil nurse, I am delighted with the learning styles available to all our learners in health and social care today. When I trained as an enrolled nurse in 1983, I spent 12 weeks in the school of nursing learning how to make beds with hospital corners, how to move patients around using a plastic mannequin, and how to carry out an aseptic technique, all in a classroom setting. We had no easy access to literature, no support from an educator outside of the classroom, clinical supervision was not yet developed as a concept, and during clinical placements there was very little in the way of structured learning support.

Once in the 'real environment' it was very much a baptism of fire. New procedures such as catheterisations were very much 'see one, do one'. I can remember how scary it felt to be practising on a patient without really having the full understanding of the 'what, how, and why' certain procedures were being carried out. The professional structures were very hierarchical, and it was not the norm to be able to ask too many questions as a subordinate. Thankfully, apart from my lack of confidence, my nerves, and embarrassment, no patients were harmed in the process, more through luck than judgement. However, this way of working did take its toll on me, the lack of supervision support left me carrying many unanswered questions and trauma from some clinical settings. Not long after qualifying, I took a couple of years out to recover. Once I returned to care of the elderly, I felt more able to start to learn and really develop as a nurse. I undertook my conversion to first level registered general nurse in 1996, and with the introduction of more modern technology and better support, it was thankfully quite a different experience. I am also happy to say that I am continuing to learn, develop, and grow in skills and confidence in healthcare every day since.

The requirement for our staff now is also to learn and re-learn continuously; this means having a 'growth mindset' influenced by technology advances and replacing routine interventions and tasks with new ways of working and delivering services. For example, virtual consultations, and supporting patients to self-care, all requiring different skill sets, multiple generations working together, and learning from one another to support this. Re-igniting 'supervision' models in practice is vital in providing guidance and feedback through structured and ad hoc opportunities in the workplace. It can help staff to maintain a sense of positivity and to gain the proper perspective on a situation; ultimately it helps to build personal resilience. Supervision is about sharing, showing, and giving support to help another person make progress and feel comfortable in their work. It involves making time and developing a practical structure to provide this support.

The benefits of supervision include enhanced accountability, increased feeling of support, development of professional skills, and improved efficiency. Supervision is also associated with decreased feelings of isolation and role ambiguity. Supervision is an accountable, two-way process, which supports, motivates, and enables the development of good practice for individual staff.

Collaborative Learning in Practice (CLiP^{TM}) was first introduced to me in 2014 in my role as director of nursing in a community trust. The CLiP opportunity was made possible with the positive relationships between the University of East Anglia and Health Education England and provider organisations across Norfolk and Waveney. There was great excitement and enthusiasm for the CLiP model between the university, deputy directors of nursing, and directors of nursing and a keenness to try it out – it was seen as a real opportunity to use supervision in action with a coaching approach. The whole concept particularly excited me as it is based on an empowering coaching model, where learners are encouraged to take the lead in their practice, caring for their own patient group with identified daily learning outcomes to achieve. It relies on a mixture of learners at different stages in their learning, working together, supporting, and learning from one and other in real time, with supervision by members of the clinical team and coached by any registered professional during the shift.

This way of working means that the learner is able to develop their own thinking, they are able to ask questions and problem solve with positive encouragement and support. Enabling learners to experience care in a psychologically safe way and think for themselves creates the opportunity for the most powerful growth in knowledge and confidence. As this model was embedded in my Trust as a fundamental way of learning, gaining momentum with educators and clinical environments, the quality of care and patient safety indicators demonstrably improved. I was delighted to bring students to tell their story to the board and at learning sessions so that wider staff from ward to board could hear first-hand the difference that the CLiP^{TM} model was making on the learner experience, staff experience, and ultimately the positive impact on patient care. I often think about my own experience as a learner and how much I would have benefitted from this approach in helping me to build my confidence and resilience earlier on.

I believe that CLiP is a modern, relevant, and fundamental way of learning, most of all it is empowering and has immediate benefits to learners, staff, and patients. I have no hesitation in commending this book to you.

Anna Morgan MBE, RGN, BSc, MA
Director of Workforce for the Norfolk and
Waveney Health & Care Partnership

Acknowledgements

We would like to convey enormous thanks to John Paul for his patience and detailed proof reading. Also, thank you to all the collaborators who worked with us to produce this book during this strange year where everyone was working during a pandemic that impacted everything.

Abbreviations

AP	Assistant Practitioner
CALM	Collaborative Assessment and Learning Model
CCC	CLiP Community Cluster project
CCEM	Clinical Clusters Education Model
CLIC	Collaborative Learning in Clusters
CLiP	Collaborative Learning in Practice
C-PAL	Coaching and Peer Assisted Learning
DH	Department of Health
DN	District Nurse
GP	General Practitioner
GROW	Goal, Reality, Options, Will do
HCA	Health Care Assistant
HDU	High Dependency Unit
HEE	Health Education England
HEENW	Health Education England – North West
HEI	Higher Education Institution
ICU	Intensive Care Unit
LL	Link Lecturer
LTHTr	Lancashire Teaching Hospitals NHS Foundation Trust
NDA	Nursing Degree Apprentice
NICE	National Institute of Health and Care Excellence
NLP	Neuro-Linguistic Programming
NMC	Nursing and Midwifery Council
OSCAR	Outcome, Situation, Choices and Consequences, Action, Review
PA	Practice Assessor

RCN	Royal College of Nursing
RePAIR	Reducing Pre-registration attrition and Improving Retention study
RN	Registered Nurse
SEN	State Enrolled Nurse
SN	Staff Nurse
SPACE model	Situation, Physiology, Action, Cognitions, and Emotions
SSSA	Standards for Student Supervision and Assessment
TA	Transactional Analysis
TFA	Thoughts Feelings Actions
TNA	Trainee Nursing Associate
TL	Team Leader
UCLAN	University of Central Lancashire
UEA	University of East Anglia
UKCC	United Kingdom Central Council for nursing and midwifery and health visiting
WHO	World Health Organisation

About the Companion Website

The book is accompanied by a website:

www.wiley.com/go/lobo/collaborativelearninginpractice

The website features:

- figures in PowerPoint format
- tables in PDF format
- learning logs
- audio clips.

Introduction

Kenda Crozier, Charlene Lobo and Rachel Paul

The Collaborative Learning in Practice (CLiP™) model is based on an established model of learning in practice used at VU University Medical Centre Amsterdam (VUmc), known as the Real-Life Learning Ward. It was developed in 2013/14 by the University of East Anglia School of Health Sciences in collaboration with NHS Practice Education Partners and NHS Health Education East of England (HEEoE). The model has subsequently been adopted, adapted, and modified by a range of organisations throughout the country.

There are two main aims of this book. First, to share our collective experiences of developing and implementing CLiP and offer others insights into our learning; and second, to offer supervisors, assessors, and students an opportunity to share the coaching skills and approaches we advocate in CLiP and to be able to use the book to support their professional development.

In producing this book, we have worked collaboratively with organisations, educators, and practitioners across the country who we feel have adhered closely to the CLiP model, using their case studies and examples of good practice to explore the model in detail. The companion website houses further examples of practice, implementation templates, and examples of assessments of learning logs and student learning journeys to be used as a development guide for the implementation of CLiP in higher education institutions (HEIs) and healthcare organisations as well as for personal development of supervisors, assessors, and students in practice who wish to develop their coaching skills.

Collaborative Learning in Practice: Coaching to Support Student Learners in Healthcare,
First Edition. Charlene Lobo, Rachel Paul, and Kenda Crozier.
© 2021 John Wiley & Sons Ltd. Published 2021 by John Wiley & Sons Ltd.
Companion website: www.wiley.com/go/lobo/collaborativelearninginpractice

In writing this book we have been faced with a major paradox in that on the one hand we advocate that coaching philosophy is a major underpinning of the model, and on the other we advocate assessing student competence in order to enable autonomous practice. A coaching purist would be aghast at the notion and might argue that the two were incompatible. Thus, from our perspective, we contend that we use coaching skills and approaches to make teaching and learning even more powerful.

At the time of development of the CLiP model, the United Kingdom (UK) Standards for Learning and Assessment in Practice (Nursing and Midwifery Council 2008) underpinned the regulatory adherence. Since then, the standards have changed, and we have attempted to highlight explicitly how the CLiP model meets the current UK regulatory standards (Nursing and Midwifery Council 2018).

In our experience, the use of the CLiP model has been in placements that are generally 6–12 weeks long. However, it has also been used successfully for rotational placements – though we would highlight the need for attention to maintaining patient and student safety in offering opportunities for students to practise autonomously where they find themselves frequently in novice situations. Thus, we advocate that the use of daily learning logs are key to ensuring safe practice for both students and patients.

PART 1 explores the current position of practice learning in nursing and midwifery in the United Kingdom. It presents the theoretical basis of the CLiP model of practice learning and the implementation of it.

Chapter 1 examines the changing context of healthcare education, the background of CLiP, and presents the case for the adoption of coaching as a learning and teaching methodology to support practice learning.

Chapter 2 provides a background literature from UK, Australia, and other countries. We explore models that have been researched nationally and internationally. The lessons learned from mentorship in the UK, practice education roles and collaborative clusters, and dedicated education units are explored to provide context to the coaching model that is the focus of this book.

Chapter 3 presents the theoretical underpinnings of the CLiP model. There are learning activities offered as questions for you to think about if you wanted to develop CLiP in your organisation/department and examples of how this has been achieved in practice. It is suggested that you collate any notes you make in answer to these questions to be used as evidence of learning for professional development. The accompanying website houses further discussion and examples of the issues raised.

Chapter 4 focuses on the organisational domain, collaborating with national partners, and presenting how CLiP was implemented at strategic, organisational, and disciplinary levels with tips and indicators on lessons learned.

Chapter 5 considers the domain of coaching as a philosophy underpinning CLiP, explicitly outlining some of the theories of coaching and how they impact on learning – with several learning activities and directed further reading to help supervisors and assessors consider how they might adopt coaching strategies to support their practice. As *educators* of nursing, midwifery, and nurse associate programmes, at the end of each discussion on coaching theory there are some points to think about in your teaching and learning practice, using coaching models and theory. As *student nurses and midwives,* you are required to develop skills in supporting and assessing your colleagues, and so we have included some tips for you in developing coaching related skills.

Chapter 6 presents evaluative studies of CLiP carried out in different organisations in England. These aim to demonstrate the current knowledge on implementation of the model and what requires further research. These are drawn from the work of research teams and signposts their published work on the topic.

PART 2 uses a case study approach to explore CLiP in action. The case studies, written in collaboration with practice partners, are all based on real-life scenarios but have been altered and adapted to ensure anonymity and highlight specific issues covered. Each chapter is focused on a case study set in a specific setting. Within each case study there are several scenarios that highlight a range of issues that may occur in the clinical setting and the approach used in the CLiP model to manage the situation. Each scenario is organised into:

 Things to think about: here is an opportunity for you to think about and make notes on how you might approach the situation. This could be an actual experience or a hypothetical proposal on how you might manage such a situation.

Applying theory to practice: discussion on how a coaching approach might apply in this scenario.

 Exemplar of a coaching conversation: signposting the theory and framework of different coaching conversations.

 Self-learning: this offers an opportunity for you to reflect on your current practice position and what you could do to become an even more powerful coach.

The aim of this part is to enable supervisors, assessors, and students to use this book to support learning and develop their coaching practice. We would encourage practitioners to keep their notes and use them as evidence for learning and professional update. Chapter 7 provides an introduction to Part 2, and is followed by Chapter 8: 'A Coaching Day', Chapter 9: Acute Hospital Ward Case Study, Chapter 10: Community Nursing Case Study, Chapter 11: Maternity Case Study, and Chapter 12: Mental Health Case Study. The Conclusion draws together the current position and looks to the future.

References

Nursing and Midwifery Council (2008). Standards to support learning and assessment in practice. NMC standards for mentors, practice teachers and teachers. NMC London https://www.nmc.org.uk/standards-for-education-and-training/standards-to-support-learning-and-assessment-in-practice/ (accessed 30 November 2020).

Nursing and Midwifery Council (2018) Standards for student supervision and assessment. https://www.nmc.org.uk/standards-for-education-and-training/standards-for-student-supervision-and-assessment/ (accessed 2 December 2020).

Glossary

Academic assessor	The academic assessor works with the practice assessor to make judgements on student progression at various stages of the programme as decided by the HEI.
Academic Link	The academic link, sometimes referred to as link lecturer, is usually a member of the higher education institution (HEI), supporting the clinical area with student and assessment concerns. They support the training of coaches and the rest of the clinical team in practice and attend the case study presentations. They also participate in the HEI role in for the preparation of students for practice.
Clinical educator	The clinical educator is an experienced clinician with enhanced teaching and assessment skills and experience to be able to support the coaches, named practice assessors, and students in practice. In the CLiP model, the clinical educator is employed by the NHS Trust or service provider and therefore understands the organisational culture and is able to support the ward/team manager in establishing CLiP as a learning culture in the practice area. One clinical educator may oversee between two to four wards areas. They also collaborate closely with the higher education link in developing and supporting practice areas.
Coach	The coach as a registered nurse, midwife, or healthcare professional will have allocated patients to care for but divides the care between the students that are being coached, allocating patients commensurate with the level and competence of the student. The coach's only responsibility for the shift should be the supervision of students.
Coachee	This coaching term applies to students or colleagues being coached. This may be student to student or supervisor to supervisor/clinical educator/link lecturer/academic link lecturer.
Practice assessor	Students have a named practice assessor who is responsible and accountable for their assessment in practice; the practice assessor may well be acting as the coach for a shift but there is no expectation by the Nursing and Midwifery Council that they will have worked substantially with a student. The practice assessor is able to make judgements about the student's practice, evidenced by the collation of daily learning logs and communication with practice supervisors which are made available for the practice assessor to review as necessary.
Practice supervisor	This refers to the registered professional supervising students in practice. Although technically a different role, it may be used interchangeably with 'mentor'.

Part I

Evolution of CLiP™

1

Changes in Practice Learning
Kenda Crozier and Charlene Lobo

Regulation of Nurse and Midwifery Education

The World Health Organization declared 2020 the year of the Nurse and Midwife and in December 2019 the Nursing and Midwifery Council (NMC) acknowledged 100 years of nursing registration in the United Kingdom. The model of hospital based 'training' of nursing, and the instigation of a register for qualified nurses in the 1919 Nurses Act, may have been the beginning of the professionalisation of nurses, but according to Davies (1977) it was also responsible for nursing shortages by restricting training places. In the century that followed we have seen changes to the Nurses and Midwives Act, the 'training' evolving from hospital control into higher education, and the registration of nurses moving from the responsibility of the General Nursing Council to the United Kingdom Central Council (with four country boards) to the current Nursing and Midwifery Council. The 1902 Midwives Act (England and Wales) established the Central Midwives Board to oversee the education and practice of midwives, thus beginning the route to professionalisation of midwifery. Today, nurses and midwives in UK practice under rules laid down in government legislation in the Health Act 1999 (UK) and Nursing and Midwifery Order 2001 (UK)[1] and subsequent amendments as statutory instruments. The need to educate more nurses to replace an ageing workforce and the requirement for

1 The Nursing and Midwifery Order 2001 (SI 2002/253).

Collaborative Learning in Practice: Coaching to Support Student Learners in Healthcare, First Edition. Charlene Lobo, Rachel Paul, and Kenda Crozier.
© 2021 John Wiley & Sons Ltd. Published 2021 by John Wiley & Sons Ltd.
Companion website: www.wiley.com/go/lobo/collaborativelearninginpractice

clinical practice experience to support this poses a difficult problem for educators to reconcile.

Throughout the early part of the twentieth century, nursing education was in the control of hospital matrons and followed the principles of Florence Nightingale. Nursing tasks were repeated throughout the period of training to demonstrate competence and to ensure that nurses understood the servitude required of their role. In the 1940s, the Wood Committee Report sought to change nurse training by recommending recognition of the student status of nurses in training. It recommended larger nursing schools and a more academic syllabus. Both the General Nursing Council and the Royal College of Nursing were concerned over the continued ability of students to contribute to the staffing of hospitals during their training (Davies 1977) and resisted the recommendations. This concern was heightened with the introduction of free healthcare via the National Health Service in 1948 which increased demand on service. From the 1940s until the 1990s, a second tier nursing qualification known as the enrolled nurse existed in support of the registered nurse (RN). The enrolled nurse training was two years long as opposed the three year RN training (Seccombe et al. 1997).

In many ways the process of practice education in clinical and care settings is a means of socialising students into the 'ways of being' a nurse, midwife, or other health professional. This phenomenon was described in the 1950s by Williams and Williams (1959) in the USA. They described three processes for socialising students including: selfless service, scientific knowledge, and authoritarian control to produce nurses. This process of behaviour modification to achieve the required social norms largely served as the means to train nurses throughout much of the first part of the twentieth century. In the second half of the twentieth century, nursing students were still expected to work alongside qualified practitioners adapting to the required behaviour and attitudes to meet the outcomes of programmes; however, there was increased emphasis on scientific knowledge and research and rather less concern with emulating and modelling selfless service.

The 1972 Briggs (Department of Health and Social Security 1972) Report made major recommendations for the separation of nurse education from service, advocating an academic degree route into nursing. There was a distinction made between the caring role of nursing and the curing role of medicine. Nurses were deemed responsible for the physical, psychological, and social health of the patient. The model of nurse education changed following the Nurses, Midwives and Health Visitors Act of 1979, from apprenticeship to education with a two part programme: an 18 month foundation followed by a further 18 months of practical training leading to registration. The disease focused, theoretical education was supported by time in the clinical environment on hospital wards where students could practise their nursing skills under the supervision of ward staff. The programme was no longer controlled by hospital matrons and clinical teachers began to appear on the wards to support student learning.

In 1983, the United Kingdom Central Council for Nursing, Midwifery and Health Visiting was created, and nurses were enabled to register in four branches as registered general nurses (RGN), registered mental health nurses (RMN), registered learning disability nurses, or registered sick children's nurses. The intention was to streamline a very unwieldy register with many different parts.

Throughout the 1980s, concern was growing about nursing shortages, the low numbers of qualified nurses being produced in the UK, and the need to recruit nurses from overseas to fill vacancies. The Royal College of Nursing identified concern about high rates of attrition from nursing programmes and recommended Project 2000 as a way forward in which students would be supernumerary in the clinical environment and the emphasis was on learning and development of skills and knowledge (Rye 1985; United Kingdom Central Council 1986). Nursing schools moved from hospitals into higher education institutions, thus emphasising the separation from service. In 1999, the Department of Health (DH) reported on further changes for nurse education in a review of the role of nurses promising a growth in recruitment, better quality placements, and better support for students in practice (Department of Health, 1999).

The training of second level enrolled nurses was phased out during the 1980s and 1990s. Seccombe et al. (1997) reported to the United Kingdom Central Council (UKCC) on confusion over role boundaries between enrolled nurses and RNs and the difficulties for those who wished to convert to RN status. Over 80% of employers reported that where nurses did convert to RN, their grade and role did not change. The phasing out of enrolled nurses saw the more widespread introduction of health-care assistants who received varying degrees of training for their role. The Willis Report (2015) identified that there were approximately 1 million healthcare assistants in the NHS supporting the work of around 330 000 RNs.

Globally, there has been a move to prepare nurses for the workforce through degree-level education. This is true for UK, Ireland and other European Union countries, USA, Australia and New Zealand, and for many on the Asian continent. This has been driven in part by changes in healthcare systems, the complexity of the health of ageing populations, and changes in the working patterns and roles of health professionals. The change from nursing apprenticeship models, where students were employed by hospitals and trained by tutors and nurses within the hospital nursing schools, to full-time degree education programmes, where students are paying for tuition and experience theoretical and practical education managed by universities, has evolved by process and policy.

In 2006, the Department of Health published 'Modernizing nursing careers' (Department of Health 2006), aimed at creating a more flexible workforce within a competency based system based on patient pathways. The nursing workforce would be presented with opportunities for career development, which could lead the changes needed in a twenty-first-century healthcare system. The report recommended raising the profile of the profession and creating clear career pathways. But it was not until 2008 that the NMC ratified plans to have an all-graduate profession of nursing by 2015, nearly 50 years after the Briggs Report. However, the concern over supply of qualified nurses into the workforce remained. The Willis Report on nurse education in 2015 made recommendations for nursing including: understanding of the role of the nurse in leading care and delegating to others; requirements for employers to properly use the graduate skills of nurses; recognition that registration on a nursing register is the beginning of a career journey; and support and provision for education and continuous professional development. The report also recommended the education of healthcare assistants leading to registration with the professional regulator. This led to the nursing associate education route being recognised by registration on the NMC register (Nursing and Midwifery Council, 2019) almost 25 years after the last enrolled nurse entered the register.

In relation to education, changes to practice education were recommended to improve quality, provide support for clinical academic careers to enable better support for students in practice settings, and to improve the evidence base for nursing education. Willis recognised the decline in nurse academic numbers and recommended that this should be reversed. Funding routes for nursing education were also singled out as an area that required urgent attention for sustainable workforce development.

The Return of the Apprentice

Recent government policy in the UK introduced a new model of apprenticeship (Nursing and Midwifery Council, 2018a,b) as a route into nursing. The model enables students to be employed by a healthcare organisation whilst on a nursing degree apprenticeship programme. The programmes are typically three or four years long. While the students on the programme are undertaking the 2300 hours of practice education, they will be supernumerary and will be released from their employment to attend theory learning. The programmes aim to encourage local recruitment to manage workforce demands, and employers have used the opportunity to develop staff who have been employed as healthcare assistants into nursing roles. This new apprentice model sits alongside the traditional university-based education with the same outcomes overseen by the regulator for nursing and midwifery nationally and is not without criticism, particularly in relation to a funding mismatch (Leary 2020). This system is similar to intern programmes in other countries identified by Budgen and Gamroth (2008). In addition, a new level of nurse, the nurse associate, has been introduced into the workforce with apprenticeship education and registration on the NMC register from 2019.

Clinical Practice Education

Successive reports into nurse education have focused on improving the quality of practice education. Securing the status of student nurses as learners rather than employees was intended to improve learning opportunities in the latter part of the twentieth century. The separation of the nursing faculty from the clinical environment has contributed to the perceived gap between theory and practice.

Learning in clinical practice has always been a critical component of student nurse education both nationally and internationally, with the quality of the clinical learning environment gaining increasing emphasis in recent years. In the UK, as elsewhere, alongside nursing shortages lies is a growing demand for clinical placements driven by greater numbers of student nurses and the decreasing availability of nurses to support learning in practice. The quality of the clinical learning environment has received further scrutiny since the Mid Staffordshire NHS Foundation

Trust Public Inquiry (Francis 2013) identified the extent of poor care in hospitals and raised questions over the quality of student learning experiences when exposed to such practice. Subsequent reports exploring nurse education, and practice learning in particular, have emphasised a need for improvement of the quality of learning environments and the quality of mentorship/supervision that supports students in practice (Willis Commission 2012, Robinson et al. 2012, Willis Report 2015, Ashton et al. 2016).

The Willis Commission (2012) identified inconsistency in the quality of practice experiences as a major concern and recognised the role of mentorship as crucial in practice education, not only in teaching, learning, and assessing but also in role-modelling good practice and leadership skills. The main barriers proposed were that mentors had insufficient time to spend with students, the increase in skill mix led to a lack of high-quality role models in practice, there was a lack of collaboration at all levels between higher education and practice that impacted on the support and training of mentors, and there was a general lack of investment in mentors and the clinical learning environment by many healthcare providers.

With increasing numbers of students and decreasing numbers of trained mentors, pressure on clinical practice areas was becoming unsustainable. In our own higher education institute (HEI), the University of East Anglia, an overview of student and mentor feedback in 2013–2014 showed mentors' commitment and the value of their role. However, a strongly emergent theme reflected 'the burden of mentorship' where mentors were faced with conflicting priorities in executing their nursing and mentoring roles, exacerbated by lack of time and increasing numbers of students. It was in this context of the realisation that one-to-one mentoring of students in practice was no longer financially or emotionally sustainable that the University of East Anglia instigated a new collaborative model based on real-life learning wards.

A subsequent review of nurse education (Willis Report 2015) identified continued inconsistencies with regard to the quality of practice learning environments but also highlighted examples of good practice, namely the Collaborative Learning in Practice (CLiP) model of practice education. The RCN (2016) commissioned a rapid review of evidence on nurse mentoring, and identified the Real-Life Learning Ward model (that originated in Amsterdam and is now running as CLiP within a UK university and

NHS partners) as one of the few models of nurse mentoring that adopted a system-wide approach. Recommendation 17 of the Willis Report (2015: p. 63) stated

> NMC should review its current mentorship model and standards, informed by the outcome of the RCN review and final evaluation of the Collaborative Learning in Practice model, and amend the standards relating to the requirement for one-to-one mentor support.

The 2018 NMC Standards for supporting student supervision and assessment do not name the model but closely advocate the main elements of the CLiP, recommending a system including practice supervisors, practice assessors, and academic assessors. It falls short of recommending a specific model of practice education leaving it to HEIs to decide this within their individual curricular models.

Establishing a Quality Learning Environment

There is a significant body of national and international literature that focuses on the quality of the clinical learning environment from both student and supervisor perspectives. Research exploring student nurse attrition has highlighted that placement experiences and the quality of support that students receive in practice can have a major impact on the student journey and significantly influence their decision to leave the course (Crombie et al. 2013, Hamshire et al. 2012). Ford et al. (2016) define quality learning environments as those that support both the students' learning and the staff that enable the learning.

There is a growing body of evidence supporting the view that quality clinical learning environments remain a complex, multifaceted phenomenon influenced by a number of interrelating factors (Jokelainen et al. 2011; Robinson et al. 2012). Predominantly, these are situated at the organisational level where they are influenced by the level of collaboration between HEIs and practice ensuring there is adequate staffing, adequate preparation of supervisors and students, adequate commitment from both organisations in relation to commitment through resources, and value placed on learning in practice (Robinson et al. 2012; Henderson and Eaton 2013). At an individual level, it centres on the relationship between the supervisor and student, whether students feel welcomed and accepted and feel the environment is safe to learn (Courtney-Pratt et al. 2012; Sandvik et al. 2014; Ford et al. 2016), and supervisors having adequate time (Robinson et al. 2012; Clements et al. 2016; Sweet and Broadbent 2017) to execute their role competently and confidently (Jokelainen et al. 2011; Henderson and Eaton 2013; Ford et al. 2016).

Against this backdrop of changes in the healthcare environment and organisational redesign of the NHS has been a reorganisation of the funding for higher education and for nursing and health profession education. Despite the assertions by the Willis Report (2015) that a long-term funding model for nursing education was needed, a system of bursary support for health profession students was withdrawn by the Department of Health and Social Care in England in 2017. This bursary had provided financial support to students of nursing and midwifery who undertook programmes with a much longer academic year (45 weeks) than the norm (30 week). Practice education requires students to experience the 24/7 nature of healthcare, so opportunities for paid employment alongside a university programme were not possible. The news of this bursary withdrawal impacted application numbers for university nursing courses and drove down student numbers. These bursaries enabled students to afford transport or accommodation to support movement across practice settings, which were a requirement of all programmes. The UK Government in 2020 announced a new NHS Learning Support Fund grant scheme for health profession students to provide financial support in recognition of the financial pressures of travelling to placements or paying dual accommodation fees during placements.

The drive for a modern healthcare profession needs to be supported by both healthcare organisations and the HEIs in a partnership that shares a vision for nursing and midwifery careers in clinical practice, policy, and in academia. There is undoubtedly a workforce shortage in the NHS and this is mirrored in academia. Taylor et al. (2010) pointed out that the career paths open to nurses need to be supported by salary scales that mean movement between clinical and academic posts is not hindered by disparity. Currently, attracting high calibre nurses into education is difficult because their earning power is greater in health organisations. The workforce issues facing the NHS are also faced by academics in higher education. Career pathways for nurses, which were identified in 'Modernizing nursing careers' (2006) need to be revisited in light of the recommendations from the Willis Report (2015).

As a final note, the planned celebrations for nursing were overtaken by the coronavirus (Covid 19) pandemic which impacted the NHS in the first six months of 2020. The NMC provided emergency standards for education and student nurses were called upon to join the NHS workforce as paid healthcare assistants while continuing their nursing education. Second- and third-year student nurses and midwives were offered the option of stepping into these new roles to continue their programmes. The supernumerary status of students was removed but learning was expected to be demonstrated. First-year students had their practice placements suspended. As we go to publication, the emergency standards are being removed, replaced by recovery standards in the process of a return to normality for nursing and midwifery education. The impact on thinking about practice-based learning has yet to be unpicked from this experience, but some concern is already being expressed (Leary 2020).

The extraordinary year in which we were producing this book reminded the world of the importance of the health workforce and particularly nursing. The impetus gained from this focus should be utilised to benefit the education of the health professions.

References

Ashton, M., Corrin, S., and Corrin, A. (2016). RCN Mentorship Project 2015. From today's support in practice to tomorrow's vision for excellence. London: RCN.

Budgen, C. and Gamroth, L. (2008). An overview of practice education models. *Nurse Education Today* 28: 273–283.

Clements, A., Kinman, G., Leggetter, S. et al. (2016). Exploring commitment, professional identity, and support for student nurses. *Nurse Education in Practice* 16: 20–26.

Courtney-Pratt, H., FitzGerald, M., Ford, K. et al. (2012). Quality clinical placements for undergraduate nursing students: a cross-sectional survey of undergraduates and supervising nurses. *Journal of Advanced Nursing* 68 (6): 1380–1390.

Crombie, A., Brindley, J., Harris, D. et al. (2013). Factors that enhance rates of completion: what makes students stay? *Nurse Education Today* 33 (11): 1282–1287.

Davies, C. (1977). Continuities in the development of hospital nursing in Britain. *Journal of Advanced Nursing* 2: 487–493.

Department of Health (1999). *Making a Difference: Strengthening the Nursing, Midwifery and Health Visiting Contribution to Health and Healthcare*. London: The Stationery Office https://webarchive. nationalarchives.gov.uk/20120504024616/http://www.dh.gov.uk/en/ Publicationsandstatistics/Publications/PublicationsPolicyAndGuidance/ DH_4007977 (accessed 30 November 2020).

Department of Health (2006). *Modernising Nursing Careers. Setting the Direction*. London: Department of Health.

Department of Health and Social Security (1972). Report of the Committee of Nursing (Chair Asa Briggs). HMSO: London

Ford, K., Courtney-Pratt, H., Marlow, A. et al. (2016). Quality clinical placements: the perspectives of undergraduate nursing students and their supervising nurses. *Nurse Education Today* 37: 97–102.

Francis, R. (2013). *Report of the Mid Staffordshire NHS Foundation Trust Public Inquiry*. London: The Stationery Office.

Hamshire, C., Willgoss, T., and Wibberler, C. (2012). 'The placement was probably the tipping point'. The narratives of recently discontinued students. *Nurse Education in Practice* 12 (4): 182–186.

Henderson, A. and Eaton, E. (2013, 2013). Assisting nurses to facilitate student and new graduate learning in practice settings: what 'support' do nurses at the bedside need? *Nurse Education in Practice* 13: 197e201.

Jokelainen, M., Turunen, H., Tossavainen, K. et al. (2011). A systematic review of mentoring nursing students in clinical placements. *Journal of Clinical Nursing* 20 (19–20): 2854–2867.

Leary, A. (2020). 'On-the-job' training takes us backwards. *Nursing Standard* 35 (8): 11–11. https://doi.org/10.7748/ns.35.8.11.s7.

Nursing and Midwifery Council (2018a). Standards framework for nursing and midwifery education Part 1 Realising professionalism: Standards for education and training. NMC: London.

Nursing and Midwifery Council (2018b). Standards framework for nursing and midwifery education Part 2: Standards for student supervision and assessment. NMC: London.

Nursing and Midwifery Council (2019). Standards for pre-registration nursing associate programmes Part 3 of Realising professionalism: Standards for education and training. NMC: London.

Robinson, S., Cornish, J., Driscoll, C., et al. (2012). Sustaining and managing the delivery of student nurse mentorship: roles, resources, standards and debates. Report for the NHS London 'Readiness for Work' programme. National Nursing Research Unit, King's College London.

Royal College of Nursing (2016). Bazian report: Rapid Evidence Review. https://www.rcn.org.uk/professional-development/publications/pub-005455 (accessed 28th February 2017).

Rye, T. (1985). The education of nurses; a new dispensation. The report of the RCN commission on nurse education. *Journal of Advanced Nursing* 1985: 10,505–10,506.

Sandvik, A., Eriksson, K., and Hilli, Y. (2014). Becoming a caring nurse – A Nordic study on students' learning and development in clinical education. *Nurse Education in Practice* 14 (3): 286–292.

Seccombe, I., Smith, G., Buchan, J., and Ball, J. (1997). *Enrolled Nurses: A Study for the UKCC*. Institute of Employment Studies.

Sweet, L. and Broadbent, J. (2017). Nursing students' perceptions of the qualities of a clinical facilitator that enhance learning. *Nurse Education in Practice* 22 (2017): 30e36.

Taylor, J., Irvine, F., Jones, C.B., McKenna, H. (2010). On the precipice of great things: the current state of UK nurse education. *Nurse Education Today* 30 (3): 239–244.

United Kingdom Central Council (1986). Project 2000: A new preparation for practice. UKCC: London.

Williams, T.R. and Williams, M.M. (1959). The socialization of the student nurse. *Nursing Research* 8 (1): 18–25.

Willis Commission (2012). *Quality with Compassion: The Future of Nursing Education*. London: The Royal College of Nursing.

Willis Report (2015). Raising the bar. shape of caring: a review of the future education and training of registered nurses and care assistants. Health Education England. https://www.hee.nhs.uk/sites/default/files/documents/2348-Shape-of-caring-review-FINAL.pdf (accessed 30 November 2020).

2

Models of Practice Learning
Kenda Crozier

Practice Education

There is a considerable body of education and nursing management literature examining models and methods of supporting nurses and other healthcare learners in clinical practice settings. There are a number of systematic reviews (Forber et al. 2016; Budgen and Gamroth 2008) on general models of practice education; the Royal College of Nursing (2015) reviewed models of mentorship and recently Williamson et al. (2020) analysed the extant evidence on collaborative learning models. This chapter therefore aims to provide a background overview of education models where support for student learning is provided within a structured approach. This includes those described in the RCN review as facilitated education models: UK mentorship and practice educator facilitation; dedicated education units; and real-life learning wards.

Developing skills and knowledge applied to the practical elements of nursing has been based on a staged approach where students begin as novices and are supported through stages of development until they demonstrate ability to perform the role of a nurse (Benner 1982, 2004) eligible for entry to a professional register.

The UK is signed up to the professional passport approach to enable professionals to work across the European Union. This agreement includes core competencies and length of programmes for nurses and

Collaborative Learning in Practice: Coaching to Support Student Learners in Healthcare,
First Edition. Charlene Lobo, Rachel Paul, and Kenda Crozier.
© 2021 John Wiley & Sons Ltd. Published 2021 by John Wiley & Sons Ltd.
Companion website: www.wiley.com/go/lobo/collaborativelearninginpractice

midwives (European Union Directive 2013/55/EU).[1] Nurse education programmes should comprise 4600 hours and at least half the programme should be in clinical practice.

> The training of nurses responsible for general care shall comprise a total of at least three years of study, which may in addition be expressed with the equivalent ECTS credits, and shall consist of at least 4600 hours of theoretical and clinical training, the duration of the theoretical training representing at least one third and the duration of the clinical training at least one half of the minimum duration of the training. (article 31 section c)

For midwives, the expectation is that clinical training should form at least one third of the programme of a total 4600 hours of theoretical and clinical education. The Nursing and Midwifery Council (NMC) expects that midwifery education should contain 4600 of which 2300 should be clinical practice (NMC 2019a).

Since 2008, UK nursing programmes are delivered at Bachelor degree level as a minimum. The higher education institutions (HEIs) must be approved by the NMC and partnered with providers of health and/or social care. The quality of care provision and by extension the quality of education provided within them is the responsibility of the partnership (NMC 2018a). The quality assurance risk assessment is part of the approval process for all new programmes of education.

The proficiency standards (NMC 2018b, 2019a) are provided to ensure a common set of outcomes that must be met at the end of a nursing or midwifery pre-registration programme anywhere in the UK. These programme outcomes are assessed through theory, practice, and simulation, but management and assessment of practice education is at the discretion of the HEIs. Clinical education is expected to take place in hospitals, community, and other settings where learners can provide care for patients or clients, and should include a range of skills acquisition and involvement in working with other professions – according to the NMC in the United

---

1 DIRECTIVE 2013/55/EU OF THE EUROPEAN PARLIAMENT AND OF THE COUNCIL of 20 November 2013 amending Directive 2005/36/EC on the recognition of professional qualifications and Regulation (EU) No. 1024/2012 on administrative cooperation through the Internal Market Information System ('the IMI Regulation').

Kingdom, which has respectively published new standards for the education of nursing students (NMC 2018a,b,c) and midwifery students (NMC 2019b).

Forber et al. (2016) explored a wide range of clinical experience models that are used internationally in nursing education. The aim of all of them is to enable development of clinical skills, although the models of nursing vary and the educational approaches differ, with many recent models including interprofessional education. The range and complexity of approaches make them difficult to study or draw meaningful comparisons from. Individual institutions and their partner organisations are therefore often in the position of taking elements of a range of models to try to plan learning for their cohorts of learners.

Practice Educator Roles

The process of becoming a nurse has long been based on role-modelling with the expectation that students learn to be nurses by working alongside nurses and developing the skills under instruction and supervision. Benner (2004), synthesising her own studies, describes the development of not only technical skills but the reasoning and critical thought required to develop and demonstrate competence and the further associated emotional engagement and moral agency that leads to expert practice. The process of supporting students to develop and demonstrate these skills and associated knowledge requires more than simply working alongside a skilled practitioner. Effective learning takes place in environments where students are not only exposed to good practice but are actively involved in care giving and challenged to make links between theory and practice. The skill mix in clinical areas means that qualified nurses are themselves working at some point on this novice to expert (Benner 2004) spectrum according to their experience of the clinical environment and patient needs. Whilst gaining and maintaining their own skills, nurses also need to consider the support of the learning needs of students, and this requires input from the HEIs. When nurses are focusing on the clinical role and responsibilities of ward management and patient care, students can be peripheral and learning ineffective (Eaton et al. 2007).

The most widely used model of practice learning is a rotational approach based on moving students around a circuit of established placements including wards, clinics, community settings, and other areas in partnerships between university or education institution and hospital or clinical setting. Budgen and Gamroth (2008) identified 10 models of clinical practice support but all involved students being placed in clinical areas for periods of time to develop skills and knowledge across different placement areas, including an increasing focus on community level nursing. Many of the models are similar or overlapping. Faculty supervised practice, joint appointments as clinical educators between universities and healthcare organisations, and secondments into roles to support students are all aimed at ensuring those supporting students have the requisite knowledge and clinical credibility. Other models may be less familiar in current UK organisations, such as internship, co-operative employment with education, work study schemes, and undergraduate nurse employment of students in their third and fourth years. These latter schemes rely on funding to employ students and the quality of education support within them is criticised (Budgen and Gamroth 2008).

Faculty and Clinical Educators in Practice Settings

The model of faculty or clinical educators supporting groups of students on wards is used widely in the USA, South East Asia, and Australia (Hunt et al. 2015; Henderson and Eaton 2013). The role of nursing faculty in the UK is now largely based in universities with oversight of quality in placement areas delivered through a link lecturer attachment to one or more clinical areas for one day per week or 20% of their teaching time. A UK study by Collington et al. (2012) explored the role of midwife academics in the practice curriculum at a time when the staff student ratio for midwifery programmes (1 : 10) differed hugely from nursing (1 : 15). Universities also received higher funding per midwifery student, linked to the greater need for midwife lecturers to be involved in clinical practice. The findings showed a variety of approaches across different institutions, including lecturers being allocated to specific maternity service providers, supporting students and staff; being linked to their personal students and supporting them in practice either through an allocation to one maternity service or by following the student placement allocation through a number of services. They also found some lecturers spent the majority of their time in practice while others visited occasionally. There were a small number of joint lecturer/practitioner appointments. Now that students are fee paying, this disparity in staff student ratio and funding no longer exists.

The clinical educator role in the UK has evolved alongside the development of models of nurse education. The role descriptor includes clinical tutor, practice placement facilitator (PPF), and practice educator. The NMC enables registration of first level nurses or midwives to record a qualification in education as lecturer/practice educator. In the 1990s, Project 2000 saw nurse education move into higher education and the role of link tutor or link lecturer evolved in response to the concerns around scaffolding students' practice experience in the new curriculum and the emphasis on higher education (Mallik and Hunt 2007). The fast pace of change was captured in a study reported by Carlisle et al. (1997) in which nurse educators described their changing role. They elucidated the tension created by attempting to balance their roles in university with an expected time commitment of one day per week in the clinical area, many describing this as only a few hours or less a week. They were regarded by their ward colleagues as no longer 'real nurses' and lacked confidence in demonstrating clinical skills. The paper predicted that university nurse educators would be involved in auditing practice learning environments, supporting the assessment of students, and providing support to clinical staff who would provide teaching to students. Carlisle et al. (1997) also predicted that the demands of a new market economy in healthcare would mean that clinical staff could not regard the support of student education as a priority. So, the tension between delivery of service to patients and clients and the education of the future workforce is not a new problem. Their recommendation for nurse practice educators with 50% role in clinical practice and 50% in higher education is still considered desirable; however, now the focus is on research and service improvement rather than education (Trusson et al. 2019). Mallik and Aylott (2005), comparing the clinical facilitator roles in UK and Australia, identified clinical credibility and cost as drawbacks to the use of these roles for support and assessment of students in practice and recommended more collaborative approaches between universities and healthcare organisations.

Mallik and Hunt (2007) evaluated a model which employed a team of practice educators to support mentors and nurses in the clinical areas. For every 50 students, 1 practice educator was in post to provide scaffolding to the learning environments through auditing and developing the learning opportunities in clinical environments. Managers and nurses perceived that the practice educators relieved some of the burden associated with supporting learners. The difficulties for some students were attributed to widening participation in nursing and recruitment of students who struggle with aspects of the programme.

Foster et al. (2015) in a mixed methods study found that students in practice negatively evaluated support from university staff. Despite requesting a link visit, students did not receive support and there appear to have been missed opportunities for link lecturers to evaluate the quality of mentorship and provide additional support to students.

McSharry et al. (2010) describes a study in Ireland that explored the role of link lecturers and clinical placement coordinators. The link lecturers lacked clinical skills and credibility and their role was characterised by infrequent contact with the clinical area. The clinical placement coordinators appeared to have stepped into this void and were perceived to provide more effective student support.

In 2003, Clarke et al. reported on an evaluation of PPF roles in three hospital environments in England. In their examination of students' views, they found positive placement experience was linked to the ward having a learning structure which ensured staff were prepared for learners; staff were valued and were interested in supporting learners; and students were supported by a mentor with whom they could work directly. The PPFs provided continuity for students as they moved between clinical areas and were used to troubleshoot issues that arose. They helped to ensure that wards were prepared for students and able to manage the learning required by signposting opportunities. However, the role of PPF, which seemed to straddle HEIs and provider hospitals, was an uncomfortable one with short-term contracts and a lack of infrastructure. Studies from Clarke et al. (2003) and Williamson and Webb (2001) demonstrated that lack of clarity in roles created insecurity not only for PPFs but also for students. Much of the short-term nature of these roles can be attributed to a lack of understanding of the educational model being enacted in the placement areas.

UK Mentorship Model

Universities and higher education institutions could not provide clinical oversight of students for the 24/7 nature of clinical practice. The NMC introduced the role of mentor into the education standards and provided guidelines for mentoring learners in practice settings (NMC 2008) – and this included a requirement for education of mentors. In the international literature, one-to-one support models for students are sometimes known as preceptorship, with mentoring considered a support mechanism for newly qualified nurses. Although attention was paid to the preparation of mentors, less emphasis was put on the organisation of clinical environments as settings for learning and this together with issues of assessment and relationships are the major criticisms of the model in the literature (Hughes et al. 2016, RCN 2015, Franklin 2013, Jokelainen et al. 2011a, Croxon and Maginnis 2009).

Mentors were expected to act as role models for students in practice and to support learning on a one-to-one basis, although the standards allowed a mentor to support up to four students (Wilkes 2006). Mentors were expected to have time for educational support activities, but often teaching time was not provided within their working day. Jokelainen et al. (2011b) demonstrated in their study that these organisational aspects of student support required greater attention from managers and those at senior level and were a source of discontentment with the mentor role.

In some cases, students simply followed a mentor and absorbed the way in which decisions were made through a process of mimicry. Although mentors had a responsibility for organising and coordinating student learning activities, in practice this was largely dependent on the clinical activity in the practice setting and also the personality and willingness of the mentor (Croxon and Maginnis 2009, Wilkes 2006, Darling 1985). Mentors were encouraged to set learning objectives to meet the outcomes documented within university produced practice assessment documents. Their role included providing written and verbal feedback and sign off on achievements during and at the end of placements and review of student portfolios linking theory and practice. This created a sense of burden on the role of mentor which increased as the number of students in clinical areas grew and numbers of mentors began to diminish (Hughes et al. 2016; Murray and Williamson 2009; Webb and Shakespeare 2008).

Hospitals and other large organisations could provide educational oversight and teams to support the allocation of students to clinical areas, but in smaller organisations the responsibility was with individual practitioners. Responsibility for quality assurance of practice learning environments was jointly held by the HEIs (universities) and the practice providers who were accountable to the regulator and to Health Education England (HEE) and its predecessors.

Quality assurance standards were tracked and quality monitoring processes included examination of organisational records to ensure that there were an adequate number of mentors to support learners. HEIs provided link lecturers to support the educational activity in practice. In effect, these lecturers oversaw quality and conducted audits of practice areas and were on hand to troubleshoot where there were concerns. On a day-to-day practical basis they were not often present (Carlisle et al. 1997) and Murray and Williamson (2009) identified that these roles suffered from a lack of clarity of definition and parity from organisation to organisation. The role of clinical educators was to a large extent phased out in many hospitals in the UK when mentorship roles were established.

The weight of responsibility for acting as gatekeepers for the profession was a heavy burden, requiring a degree of courage as well as judgement. The NMC 2008 (p. 17) stated this responsibility as:

> Mentors, practice teachers and teachers who sign off all, or part of the practice component of a programme leading to registration are accountable to the Council for their decisions.

Whilst there was the expectation of supporting learners with effective assessment, the reality was all too often that mentors sought to shape students in their own image. The aim of many students was therefore to fit in and not to stand out (Levett-Jones et al. 2009). Scholes et al. (2004) found concerns among mentors about the use of portfolios, lack of confidence, and lack of clarity in learning outcomes. Portfolios were designed to enable students to reflect on the theory and its application to practice; those with stronger writing skills found this easier and mentors' own theoretical knowledge was questionable. The time to support this activity, including interpreting the requirements and identifying material, was also a distraction from the clinical aspects of learning and doing. Webb and Shakespeare (2008), using Benner's decision making as a basis to interview mentors, found that making a judgement on student performance was based on good mentoring, good students, and good mentoring relationships. They reiterated findings from Scholes et al. (2004) that greater support for mentors was needed particularly when concerns about student progress were an issue, and there were requirements for mandatory attendance at updates, greater emphasis on time and status for the mentor role, as well as greater attention to student evaluations of mentoring and placement settings. The Willis (2012) Commission echoed the view that mentorship models were not effective due to their lack of status and support.

The relationship between individual mentors and students did produce pressure on mentors to pass students. The concepts underpinning mentoring were sound but the practical relationship between mentors and learners was fraught with difficulties, including the much debated issue of 'failure to fail' (Hughes et al. 2016). Harrison-White and Owens (2018) found that one of the key challenges for students was fitting in with the ways of working of mentors in busy clinical environments. Where learning opportunities were blocked due to power dynamics or other issues, students adopted a survival mode in order to complete the placement or formed alliances with HCAs and adopted their ways of working. Link lecturers in this study were interviewed in focus groups and expressed concern about the power dynamics and clinical demands in practice settings, but there appeared to be little reflection on their own roles in mediating these learning relationships and certainly no consideration of them using opportunities for teaching in practice. The authors of this paper allude to the new NMC Standards (2018a,b,c) and the need for cooperation between academic and practice assessors, and are cautious about the need for there to be more capacity in clinical environments to accommodate student learning. As written, the new standards do not address how this capacity can be built in.

Hub and Spoke Models

Astley-Cooper (2012) suggested that a hub and spoke model would enable students to take control of their own learning, and access relevant experiences within a wider community of practice in order to understand the bigger picture of patient care. Many curriculum models used the hub and spoke approach supported by clinical educators but encountered difficulties with issues of capacity and planning. Problems also arose with providing continuity of mentorship within the model to meet the NMC requirement that a mentor should be available to the student for

40% of the placement time. Roxburgh (2011) found that students liked a mixture of hub and spoke that allowed for a main placement base with secure mentorship in year 1 with the option of rotational placements in year 2, when they felt more confident in their approach to practice. Thomas and Westwood (2016) evaluated the hub and spoke model used in practice learning, finding that the purpose of the spoke elements was not always clear to students. Coordination of learning in the spokes was lacking and therefore the value of learning was sometimes lost if the spokes were not well planned within the placement framework. The hubs contributed to the sense of belongingness previously identified as important by Levett-Jones et al. (2009), but this depended on the quality of mentorship.

The Student Perspective

So, it is very important that we turn our attention to understanding the experience of learners in the practice placement environments. Student satisfaction with programmes is deeply connected to the support and learning they experience in clinical practice environments. The Health Education England RePAIR (Health Education England 2018) report found attrition from nursing programmes is associated with poor experiences in practice learning environments.

Gray and Smith's (2000) longitudinal study of student nurses examined their view of mentor qualities. Students described dependence on the mentor growing more distant in the later part of their programme. The qualities they valued were those of support, guidance, and knowledgeable clinical expertise.

Levett-Jones et al. (2009) report that the importance of fitting in and being part of the team was linked by students to an ability to develop the skills needed to grow as nurses. Simply feeling welcome in an environment was a high-level motivator for students. However, they reported contradictory experiences in wanting to be given autonomy as third-year students but experiencing a sense of heightened expectations about their competence which they could not deliver. Staff who provided consistent support enabled growth of confidence, whilst being ignored or undervalued left students unable to fulfil their potential. This Australian study examined the nursing staff as a whole rather than focusing only on those providing a mentorship or teaching role, recognising that the wider staff have a contributing role in student learning.

Jack et al. (2018) surveyed student nurses, finding that learners felt neglected or were subjected to unfair treatment by clinical staff. The mentor role designed to support them did not work when allocated mentors were on leave, which meant students felt cut adrift. In addition, they reported that the supernumerary status of students was not respected and they were regarded as another 'pair of hands' in the workforce. Students were torn between wanting to feel that they were part of a team but also being treated as learners and supported to develop their knowledge and skills in a safe way. The study exemplifies some of the concern that was being raised among academics and clinicians about the mentor role. It also demonstrates the tensions between 'learning through doing' and having supernumerary status.

Likewise, students expressed concern about mentors who neglected or bullied them (Jack et al. 2018). They reported feeling 'outsiders' and being undermined and anxious, creating barriers to learning (Astley-Cooper 2012). The workload of registered nurses was concerned with coordinating and managing care whilst the students they supervised were responsible for delivering individual care. Therefore, the role-modelling students expected to find did not exist. Often students existed in a space between the qualified nurses and the healthcare assistants. They received instruction from both and felt this division of workload impeded their ability to see and experience the nursing care they were expected to provide once qualified (Astley-Cooper 2012). The students therefore did not work alongside their mentors and saw that the expected learning outcomes did not relate to the role performed by qualified nurses. They therefore questioned the need for the learning they were undertaking, as once qualified they would be performing the coordination and management roles rather than providing hands-on care. The students again reported a sense of feeling of being 'used as a pair of hands' (Astley-Cooper 2012: p. 147). Students saw good mentoring as planning the learning with a logical sequence to support the development of skills towards the learning outcomes. Students did not always experience learning in a sequence that made sense to them.

McIntosh et al. (2013) explored the experiences of third-year students on midwifery programmes in six UK universities. They found that students identified dissonance between the discursive critical thinking approach to the theoretical elements of the programme and the practice experience during which there appeared to be a finite set of dexterous skills and knowledge to be gained and demonstrated. Students felt unprepared for their practical role due to the tension between these two elements of their education. This is similar to the experience Philpin reported in 1999 and to the findings from Astley-Cooper (2012) who reported the lack of importance placed on higher order thinking skills in clinical practice. Philpin (1999) reported tension between the idealised approach to nursing presented by educators and the bureaucratic reality of the experience of nursing in clinical practice. This theory–practice gap is an ongoing challenge, yet the need for higher order skills of critical thinking and clinical leadership were made inherent in the Department of Health vision for modern nursing in 2006.

The RePAIR report (Health Education England 2018) on student attrition identified that support in the clinical environment was a key factor impacting student decisions to leave programmes. Poor communication between education institutions and healthcare providers meant that the expectations of students was confused. The support of mentors and practice educators could influence a student's experience of learning in both positive and negative ways.

Dedicated Education Units and Clinical Clusters

New models of practice learning support have been developed in Australia in response to nurse shortages and the need to increase placement capacity for students. The previous model of dedicated education units, developed in the 1990s, is widely used in Australia and South East Asia and also in the USA (Grealish et al. 2018; Hunt et al. 2015, Henderson and Eaton 2013).

Dedicated education units were described by Wotton and Gonda (2004) as 'existing health care units collaboratively developed by clinicians and academics as clinical teaching and learning environments dedicated to students'. The aim of setting up the units was to develop the relationship between universities and clinical areas to improve the learning experiences of students. Student nurses in the units came from three separate education institutions, so previous problems of expectations and learning needs had been identified because of the different organisations involved. The partnership approach included students from all year groups working together supported by nurses and academics to develop clinical competence. The model worked through students having two days in the clinical environment, two days in university, and one day personal study per week (Wotton and Gonda 2004). This sits alongside other more traditional block placements that do not contain university time. The evaluation of students and clinicians identified strong relationships and peer-to-peer support among students. There were also improved collaborative relationships between academics and clinicians with the exception of some confusion about who should be responsible for the development of students. Third-year students were more likely to find the combined academic and clinical workload stressful. The clinicians indicated that they were supported in clinical teaching but that they needed further education and support to develop their skills.

This innovative curriculum model relies on academics having clinical confidence and a workload balance that enables this degree of time in practice. The faculty role in the US also supports this model, with academics expected to maintain their clinical expertise through regular clinic or ward practice (Hunt et al. 2015).

Henderson et al. (2006) used a clinical learning environment inventory to assess students' perceptions of the psychosocial aspects of the learning environment. They make a powerful case for the presence of a clinical facilitator to support nurses in wards where students are placed. The clinical facilitator enables discussion and reflection on practice and develops critical thinking linking theory and practice. This benefits not only students but also the staff supporting their learning.

Henderson and Eaton (2013) reported on the support of preceptors (nurses supporting the development of learners and new graduates) through monthly updates as a precursor to the development of a new model of collaborative education. This model of nurses being provided with educational theory to enable them to support workplace learning and assessment seems similar to the mentorship approach used in the UK. The development of preceptor models came as a precursor to Clinical Clusters Education Model (CCEM) used by Grealish and colleagues in Australia, which enables students to work with nurses in clinical areas whilst also having access to supported facilitation by a clinical educator. The co-designed model of learning was implemented using a structured and supported approach that considered the feasibility issues of the model (Grealish et al. 2018). In the mixed methods evaluation of CCEM, it was found that the mix of nurses supporting learners with the encouragement and development offered by clinical facilitators (known in the model as 'entry to practice facilitators') improved learning opportunities for students and provided better integration of learners within the clinical setting. However, there was some confusion over roles and students were unsure of who was assessing and providing feedback at times. Nurses require further support to enable the process of identifying learning opportunities and continuous feedback to students to be effective for learning (van de Mortel et al. 2020). In the model, peer discussion groups in which students shared learning facilitated by clinical educators supported the link between theory and practice. Van de Mortel et al. (2020) report on an observational study of these learning circles where students were encouraged to discuss a clinical situation using a concept mapping approach. Although the facilitators had been trained in the new methods, they sometimes reverted to their traditional discussion group style. The groups only met once so the evaluation could not sufficiently discover the value of a longer term set of meetings over time for student learning. The CCEM model shows promise but also identifies the difficulties of transitioning between models of practice education.

Real-Life Learning Wards

The real-life learning ward is similar to the dedicated education unit, enabling students to enact the roles they are being prepared for in a real-life environment, and was aimed originally at third-year students. The original concept was developed by Wahlstrom and Sanders (1998) in Linkoping, Sweden as part of an interprofessional learning module culminating in two weeks practice on an orthopaedic ward where final-year students from nursing, medicine, physiotherapy, and other programmes provided patient care under supervision. In the approach used in Sweden, faculty members oversaw the students working on the ward. The model has been adopted and adapted by others, where staff numbers are those required to deliver the care on a shift and students are supernumerary. The students take a problem-based approach to their learning and are effectively providing the care. This level of responsibility prepares students for their role as qualified practitioners

(Freeth et al. 2001; Hellstrom-Hyson et al. 2012). Comparing the model to traditional supervision in practice placements, students felt more confident in the student-led wards, they took responsibility and found they were able to fulfil the role supported by their peers. However, they felt undermined and lost confidence when the supervising nurse took over care (Hellstrom-Hyson et al. 2012).

The range of models of practice education are varied with different measures applied to the published studies so the process of drawing comparisons is not easy. In this chapter, we have provided an overview of some of the commonly used approaches that have been applied in the UK. It is within this mixed context of care provision and education that we place the Collaborative Learning in Practice model.

References

Astley-Cooper, J. (2012). The lived experience of student nurses in clinical placement. Unpublished PhD thesis. University of Swansea.

Benner, P. (1982). From novice to expert. *American Journal of Nursing* 82: 402–407.

Benner, P. (2004). Using the Dreyfus model of skill acquisition to describe and interpret skill acquisition and clinical judgement in nursing practice and education. *Bulletin of Science, Technology & Society* 24 (3): 188–199.

Budgen, C. and Gamroth, L. (2008). An overview of practice education models. *Nurse Education Today* 28: 273–283.

Carlisle, C., Kirk, S., and Luker, K.A. (1997). The clinical role of nurse teachers within a project 2000 course framework. *Journal of Advanced Nursing* 25: 386–395.

Clarke, C.L., Gibb, C.E., and Ramprogus, V. (2003). Clinical learning environments: an evaluation of an innovative role to support preregistration nursing placements. *Learning in Health and Social Care* 2 (2): 105–115.

Collington, V., Mallik, M., Doris, F., and Fraser, D. (2012). Supporting the midwifery practice based curriculum: the role of the link lecturer. *Nurse Education Today* 32 (2012): 924–929.

Croxon, L. and Maginnis, C. (2009). Evaluation of clinical teaching models for nursing practice. *Nurse Education in Practice* 9 (4): 236–243.

Darling, L.A. (1985). What to do about toxic mentors. *Journal of Nursing Administration* 15 (5): 43–44.

Eaton, E., Henderson, A., and Winch, S. (2007). Enhancing nurses' capacity to facilitate learning in nursing students: effective dissemination and uptake of best practice guidelines. *International Journal of Nursing Practice* 13: 316–332.

Forber, J., DiGiacomo, M., Carter, M. et al. (2016). In pursuit of an optimal model of undergraduate nurse education: an integrative review. *Nurse Education in Practice* 21: 83–92.

Foster, H., Ooms, A., and Marks-Maran, D. (2015). Nursing students' expectations and experiences of mentorship. *Nurse Education Today*: 18–24.

Franklin, N. (2013, 2013). Clinical supervision in undergraduate nursing students: a review of literature. *E- Journal Business Education and Scholarship of Teaching.* 7 (1): 34–42.

Freeth, D., Reeves, S., Goreham, C. et al. (2001, 2001). 'Real life' clinical learning on an interprofessional training ward. *Nurse Education Today* 21: 366–372.

Gray, M.A. and Smith, L.N. (2000). The qualities of an effective mentor from the student nurse's perspective: findings from a longitudinal qualitative study. *Journal of Advanced Nursing* 32 (6): 1542–1549.

Grealish, L., van de Mortel, T., Brown, C. et al. (2018). Redesigning clinical education for nursing students and newly qualified nurses: a quality improvement study. *Nurse Education in Practice* 2018: 84–89.

Harrison-White, K. and Owens, J. (2018). Nurse link lecturers' perceptions of the challenges facing student nurses in clinical learning environments: a qualitative study. *Nurse Education in Practice* 32: 78–83.

Health Education England (2018). RePAIR Report. Reducing pre-registration attrition and improving Retention.

Hellstrom-Hyson, E., Martensson, G., and Kristofferzon, M. (2012). To take responsibility or to be an onlooker. Nursing students' experiences of two models of supervision. *Nurse Education Today* 32: 105–110.

Henderson, A. and Eaton, E. (2013, 2013). Assisting nurses to facilitate student and new graduate learning in practice settings: what 'support' do nurses at the bedside need? *Nurse Education in Practice* 13: 197e201.

Henderson, A., Twentyman, M., Heel, A., and Lloyd, B. (2006). Students' evaluation of the impact of clinical education units on psycho- social aspects of the clinical learning environment. *Australian Journal of Advanced Nursing* 23: 8–13.

Hughes, L.J., Mitchell, M., and Johnston, A.N.B. (2016). 'Failure to fail' in nursing- a catch phrase or a real issue? A systematic integrative literature review. *Nurse Education in Practice* 20: 54–63.

Hunt, D., Milani, M.F., and Wilson, S. (2015). Dedicated education units. An innovative model for clinical education. *American Nurse Today* 10 (5): 46–49.

Jack, K., Hamshire, C., Harris, W.E. et al. (2018). "My mentor didn't speak to me for the first four weeks": perceived unfairness experienced by student nurses in clinical practice settings. *Journal of Clinical Nursing* 27: 929–993.

Jokelainen, M., Turunen, H., Tossavainen, K. et al. (2011a). A systematic review of mentoring nursing students in clinical placements. *Journal of Clinical Nursing* 20 (19–20): 2854–2867.

Jokelainen, M., Jamookeeah, D., Tossavainen, K., and Turunen, H. (2011b, 2011). Building organizational capacity for effective mentorship of pre-registration nursing students during placement learning: Finnish and British mentors' conceptions. *International Journal of Nursing Practice* 17: 509–517I.

Levett-Jones, T., Lathlean, J., Higgins, I., and McMillan, M. (2009). Staff student relationships and their impact on nursing students' belongingness and learning. *Journal of Advanced Nursing* 65 (2): 316–324.

Mallik, M. and Aylott (2005). Facilitating practice learning in pre-registration nursing programmes – a comparative review of the Bournemouth collaborative model and Australian models. *Nurse Education in Practice* 5: 152–160.

Mallik, M. and Hunt, J.A. (2007). Plugging a hole and lightening the burden: a process evaluation of a practice education team. *Journal of Clinical Nursing* 16: 1848–1857.

McIntosh, T., Fraser, D.M., Stephen, N., and Avis, M. (2013). Final year students' perceptions of learning to be a midwife in six British universities. *Nurse Education Today* 33: 1179–1183.

McSharry, E., McGloin, H., Frizzel, A.M., and Winters-O'Donnell, L. (2010). The role of nurse lecturer in clinical practice in the Republic of Ireland. *Nurse Education in Practice* 10: 189–195.

Murray, S.C. and Williamson, G.R. (2009). Managing capacity issues in clinical placements for pre-registration nurses. *Journal of Clinical Nursing* 18: 3146–3154.

Nursing and Midwifery Council (2008). Standards to support learning and assessment in practice. NMC standards for mentors, practice teachers and teachers. NMC London. https://www.nmc.org.uk/standards-for-education-and-training/standards-to-support-learning-and-assessment-in-practice/ (accessed 30 November 2020).

Nursing and Midwifery Council (2018a). Programme standards: standards for pre-registration nursing programmes. https://www.nmc.org.uk/standards/standards-for-nurses/standards-for-pre-registration-nursing-programmes/ (accessed 30 November 2020).

Nursing and Midwifery Council (2018b). Standards of proficiency for registered nurses. https://www.nmc.org.uk/standards/standards-for-nurses/standards-of-proficiency-for-registered-nurses/ (accessed 30 November 2020).

Nursing and Midwifery Council (2018c). *Standards Framework for Nursing and Midwifery Education Part 1 Realising Professionalism: Standards for Education and Training* NMC London. https://www.nmc.org.uk/standards-for-education-and-training/standards-framework-for-nursing-and-midwifery-education/ (accessed 30 November 2020).

Nursing and Midwifery Council (2019a). Realising professionalism: Standards for education and training. Part 3: standards for pre-registration midwifery programmes. https://www.nmc.org.uk/globalassets/sitedocuments/standards/standards-for-pre-registration-midwifery-programmes.pdf (accessed 30 November 2020).

Nursing and Midwifery Council (2019b). Standards of proficiency for midwives. https://www.nmc.org.uk/globalassets/sitedocuments/standards/standards-of-proficiency-for-midwives.pdf (accessed 30 November 2020).

Philpin, S.M. (1999). The impact of project 2000 educational reforms on the occupational socialisation of nurses: an exploratory study. *Journal of Advanced Nursing* 29 (6): 1326–1331.

Roxburgh, M. (2011). Undergraduate student nurses' perceptions of two practice learning models: a focus group study. *Nurse Education Today* 34 (2014): 40–46.

Royal College of Nursing (2015). Nurse mentoring: Rapid evidence review. A report for the Royal College of Nursing. RCN London.

Scholes, J., Webb, C., Gray, M. et al. (2004). Making portfolios work in practice. *Journal of Advanced Nursing* 46: 595–603.

Thomas, M. and Westwood, N. (2016). Student experience of the hub and spoke model of placement allocation – an evaluative study. *Nurse Education Today* 46: 24–28.

Trusson, D., Rowley, E., and Bramley, L. (2019, 2019). A mixed methods study of challenges and benefits of clinical academic careers for nurses, midwives and allied health professionals. *BMJ Open* 9: e030595. https://doi.org/10.1136/bmjopen-2019-030595.

Van de Mortel, T., Armit, L., Shenahan, B. et al. (2020). Supporting Australian clinical learners in a collaborative clusters education model: mixed methods study. *BMC Nursing* 19: 57.

Wahlstrom, O. and Sanden, I. (1998). Multiprofessional training ward at Linkoping university: early experience. *Education for Health: Change in Learning & Practice* 11 (2): 225–231.

Webb, C. and Shakespeare, P. (2008, 2008). Judgements about mentoring relationships in nurse education. *Nurse Education Today* 28: 563–571.

Wilkes, Z. (2006). The student-mentor relationship: a review of the literature. *Nursing Standard* 20 (37): 42–47. https://doi.org/10.7748/ns2006.05.20.37.42.c4160.

Williamson, G.R. and Webb, C. (2001). Supporting students in practice. *Journal of Clinical Nursing* 10: 284–292.

Williamson, G.R., Plowright, H., Kane, A. et al. (2020). Collaborative learning in practice: a systematic review and narrative synthesis of the research evidence in nurse education. *Nurse Education in Practice* 43 (2020): 102706.

Willis Commission (2012). *Quality with Compassion: The Future of Nursing Education*. London: The Royal College of Nursing.

Wotton, K. and Gonda, J. (2004). Clinician and student evaluation of a collaborative clinical teaching model. *Nurse Education in Practice* 4: 120–127.

3

The CLiP™ Model

Charlene Lobo and Jonty Kenward

This chapter explains the theoretical underpinning of the CLiP model of practice education. It also aims to help support the implementation of the CLiP model by offering:

 Questions for you to think about.

 Examples of how it could be implemented in practice.

 Go to the companion website which provides more in-depth discussion and examples.

NMC (2018) signposting to the particular standard of the United Kingdom Nursing and Midwifery Council (2018) Standards for Student Supervision Assessment.

The CLiP model grew out of a need to increase placement capacity without negatively impacting on the quality of the learning environment. In 2014, having changed the process of obtaining practice placement feedback, we were able to collate a significant level of feedback to conduct a comprehensive analysis of the experiences of students and mentors over the year. The overall comments from students were very positive and, although many mentors valued supporting students, a significant theme that came from mentors was the 'burden of mentoring'. Thus, for us it was clear that the current mentorship model was not viable not only in terms of the burden of mentorship, but also in its inability to deliver adequate placement capacity.

So, a journey to explore different models of practice education in nursing and midwifery began, and it was through the university's research engagement with VU Medical Centre, Amsterdam (VUmc) that we discovered a model of practice learning that was described as the 'Real-Life Learning Ward'. For us, this model of nurse education was distinct from the traditional one-to-one UK mentorship model in the way practice learning was organised and implemented – and in the coaching philosophy that underpinned how students learnt. Table 3.1 highlights the differences we found between the Real-Life Learning Ward at VUmc and the mentorship model exercised in our area with our practice partners.

The CLiP model was developed by the University of East Anglia in collaboration with its practice and commissioning partners based on the 'Real-Life Learning Ward' and the prevailing standards to support nursing and assessment in practice (NMC 2008).

The fundamental basis of the model is that care is delivered to patients by a registered nurse *through* the students, meaning that students are directly involved in hands-on patient care supervised by a 'coach' who is a registered nurse but not necessarily a mentor (NMC 2018 SSSA 1.11; 2.7). For example, on a ward the registered nurse who would be acting as 'coach' for the shift might be allocated nine patients and three students to supervise. The patient care will then be divided between the students in a negotiated and collaborative way depending on the experience, competence, capability, and learning outcomes of the students (NMC 2018 SSSA 1.7; 1.9; 1.10). At the beginning of the shift, students and their coach review the patient group they will be caring for, negotiate how the delivery of care is to be divided between the students, the level of supervision and support required by each student, and work together as a team to deliver the care with the coach always available, observing, assessing, and supervising practice. Learning environments need to have access to resource facilities where students can pursue further research and study as needed in relation to the care they are assigned to deliver. Again, time off from patient care needs to be negotiated with peers and coaches to ensure patient care is always covered.

Students have a named assessor (NMC 2018 SSSA 6.2; 6.3; 6.4; 6.6) who retains responsibility of their overall practice assessment, which is based

Table 3.1 Differences between mentor model and VUmc model.

Traditional UK mentorship model	Real-life learning ward
Maximum 6–8 students per ward.	18–20 students per ward.
Usually one mentor supports one student, often one mentor and one associate mentor per student.	One coach supervises 2–4 students.
Learning is often task focused, working alongside a mentor. Sometimes more experienced students are allocated total patient care.	Students are responsible for total patient care, commensurate with competence and their level of practice.
Mentor as expert.	Coach as facilitator.
Mentor directs student learning and development, providing learning opportunities.	Students take responsibility for their own learning, negotiating learning opportunities with their coach.
Students are allocated a named mentor with the aim to achieve minimum 40% student supervision by the named mentor.	Nominated coach can vary on a daily basis.
The named mentor is responsible for the assessment of students in practice.	Students collate written assessment of competence completed by the coach in their learning logs on a daily basis.
Mentors often have a range of practice/ward responsibilities in addition to supervising students.	The coach's only responsibility for the shift is to coach students.
A high level of competing priorities for mentors impacts on the availability of time to provide contemporaneous discussion, reflection and feedback for students.	A highly structured day focusing only on the students. This enables mentors time for case reviews, team discussion, critical reflection, and immediate feedback.
An educational pedagogy underpins student supervision.	A coaching pedagogy underpins student supervision.
Occasionally a student 'buddy' approach is adopted but this is not a common model of practice.	Peer (students of the same educational level) and tiered (students at different levels, e.g. mixed first, second, and third years) learning is adopted.

on a range of evidence collated in their learning logs. These learning logs are compiled from the student's intended learning outcomes for the day with the assessment and feedback given by coaches who have supervised their practice on the shifts they have worked. The whole learning environment is facilitated by a clinical educator who is an experienced mentor whose role is to support both students and coaches in practice (NMC 2018 SSSA 1.5; 2.2). In this way, a collaborative approach to student supervision and assessment is adopted. Figure 3.1 demonstrates student support in practice.

The two main areas of difference noted between the Real-Life Learning Wards and the mentorship model were the way learning was organised and the use of coaching strategies and approaches to facilitate student learning; these two differences evolved to represent the two main domains of the CLiP model. Within these two domains we noted five themes that we felt were vital in providing a high quality of learning – collaboration, real-life learning, time to teach and time to learn, stepping up, stepping back, and assessment and feedback. These key themes evolved into a set of principles that supported the model. Further, in the implementation process we noted that these domains and principles applied across individual, practice and organisational levels which integrated to deliver a systematic approach to practice learning. Figure 3.2 represents the CLiP model of practice education.

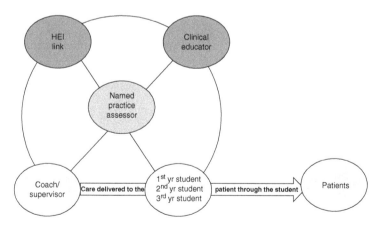

Figure 3.1 CLiP™ model of student support.

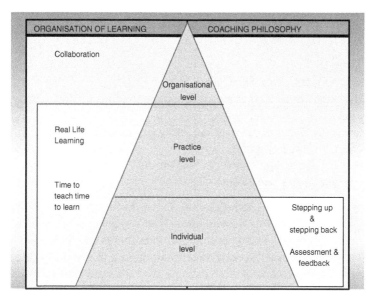

Figure 3.2   CLiP™ model.

Domains of CLiP

Organisation of Learning

A well-organised practice learning environment involves the whole team ensuring they are all prepared and trained to receive and support students and are clear about the expectations from them and from students. This level of organisation helps students feel welcome and accepted, which are well established as critical aspects of high-quality clinical learning environments (Levett-Jones and Lathlean 2008; Courtney-Pratt et al. 2012) and play an important part in students feeling they have a legitimate place on the team and a right to learn (Jokelainen et al. 2013; Ford ct al. 2016). The two key organisational factors necessary for a high-quality learning environment are as follows:

i) Administrative allocation of students to practice areas.
   This requires advance planning in order to allocate the right number of students to a practice area and ensure that both students and staff have adequate notice to prepare for students starting placements.

Think about your Clinical Environment

How many patients do you have?
What range of care requirements are there in terms of high dependency/low dependency/rehabilitation?
How is the layout of the ward/department organised?
What is the ratio of staff to patients?
What might the right number of students be?
How will this be worked out?

Our 30 bedded neuro surgical ward is made up of 6 bays and 3 side rooms. This is a medium dependency unit for mainly male patients following neurosurgical procedures and high acuity. The staffing is usually one qualified staff nurse and one healthcare assistant to a maximum of 10 patients, with the ward manager and nurse in charge organising the ward on a shift by shift basis. Where required, further support is offered for the requirement of enhanced patients.

This ward takes up to 25 student nurses at any one time in the academic year. This is worked out with regards to the number of appropriately prepared qualified assessors and supervisors available to support; roughly this equates to five students to each assessor and for coaches this will depend on the learner and the size of the unit and its acuity. For example, if they are all first-year students then we would allocate between six and eight to one coach. Similarly, if there are second- and third-year students, then there might be four students allocated to a coach. The ward opens up to CLiP on a staggered basis dependant on how many students are present as our learners come out on to placement in a staggered process. They also come out in different year groups, so the allocation of learners is also dependant on the level of learner in the area.

Initially, we did not allow our students to work long days because of all the research pointing to the higher incidence of 'never' events occurring after 5 p.m. and also because we think it is too long for our learners to carry the responsibility of care for that length of time.

As we have moved through the project, we have found that we need to offer some flexibility, so students are allowed one long day/week in exceptional circumstances.

ii) The preparation of the practice team.

This involves introducing the whole team to the CLiP model of learning, equipping all supervisors (including healthcare assistants) with coaching skills and enhancing their 'pedagogical competence' as described by Jokelainen et al. (2011); i.e., the ability to competently assess students in practice. Ford et al. (2016) claim a gap exists between what students and supervisors expect from each other in terms of performance and behaviour and therefore preparation of both is important for a good placement experience. Further, our own experience has demonstrated that when the whole practice team is involved in the preparation it helps build what could be called 'engagement capital', namely increasing the practice area commitment to student learning, enhancing the students' sense of belongingness and feeling valued, and building their sense of safety and security – which are well-established factors that enhance student learning in the clinical environment (Levett-Jones and Lathlean 2008).

 Think about Preparing your Clinical Area for CLiP

Which members of the clinical team would you include?
What might this involve?
How could you logistically accomplish this?

 Example of the implementation at ward level

Our ward decided that we wanted to adopt the CLiP approach to placement and approached our hospital educational lead. A clinical educator and link lecturer supported implementation.

(Continued)

(Continued)

The implementation of CLiP was initiated by a staff briefing presentation campaign and entire multidisciplinary team involvement. A 'ward to board' cascade approach was adapted to aid this process. 'Coach the coaches' preparation consisted of one evening session by two higher education institutions (HEI) lecturers discussing 'situational leadership'. Additional coaching sessions were provided by HEI and supported by members of the ward team, which included the clinical educator, ward manager, and senior mentor. Both the clinical educator and the HEI link lecturer support the coaches from the commencement of CLiP. The clinical educator observes the coaches and facilitates ongoing coaching skills. Students have the equivalent of a one-day trust induction and departmental orientation, which includes preparation for CLiP. Students are also prepared by the HEI on campus for the CLiP experience and where possible one or two members of staff attend the preparation session, which is very useful to answer any questions students have and to demonstrate a collaborative approach between HEI and practice. Thereafter, students have a one-week orientation period on the ward where they work closely, one-to-one with a mentor.

 Go to the companion website for examples of the CLiP implementation process.

Coaching Philosophy

The coaching philosophy of CLiP is exercised predominantly through coaching strategies and approaches used by supervisors and forms the basis of the student–coach relationship. According to Rogers et al. (2012), the whole aim of coaching is to close the gap between potential and performance, to facilitate learning by enabling people to find their own solutions, develop their skills, and change their practice. This reflects the coaching philosophy of CLiP in that learning is student led, a facilitative style is adopted by supervisors to enable students to develop their own solutions to care, and questioning is used to provide critical challenge and to develop reflective decision-making skills. There is limited literature on the use of coaching approaches with undergraduate nursing and midwifery students in clinical practice. However, a study by Kelton (2014) demonstrated the successful use of a clinical coach role in supporting failing students' clinical competence.

Principles of CLiP

Within the two domains of CLiP lie five principles that are implemented at an individual, practice and organisational level.

Collaboration

Collaboration is a fundamental principle of CLiP and exists across both domains and at several levels:

- Organisational level – involving HEI, practice organisations, and commissioning partners.
- Practice level – involving the range of professionals in the team/practice area.
- Individual level – between coach and student and between students through peer learning.

At an organisational level, collaboration between academic and practice organisations is vital to ensure the quality of learning environments (Ford et al. 2016; Jokelainen et al. 2011; Henderson and Eaton 2013), a key focus being on the need for adequate preparation of supervisors to facilitate student learning and assess them in practice (Duffy 2003; Jokelainen et al. 2011; Hamshire et al. 2012; Henderson and Eaton 2013). Within the CLiP model, the role of the clinical educator and the collaboration between clinical educator and the HEI plays a key function in facilitating organisational collaboration. Henderson and Eaton (2013) advocate that collaboration across organisations at senior management level is imperative to influence a cultural change within care delivery where mentors and supervisors are protected to support students in practice, failing to do so does not value the work they do and works against legitimacy of facilitating learning in practice. We found a further consideration of collaboration at organisational level is sustaining the commitment and support, especially when champions at senior level change or move on (see concluding chapter).

Collaboration at a multiprofessional level is crucial for the whole of the ward/ practice/department team committed to real-life learning in order to create a learning environment where students engage in the real-life experience of nursing. Part of taking full responsibility of care delivery is to initiate/respond to professional conversations (albeit under supervision) with other healthcare staff such as doctors, consultants, allied health professionals, and healthcare assistants, as well as patients and their relatives. Thus, to ensure students are able to step up to this, the whole team needs to engage as part of the learning culture. Collaboration across the whole team is also necessary to ensure that the coaches' time is protected to solely focus on the supervision of students to produce a quality learning environment that creates 'time to teach and time to learn'.

Another aspect of collaboration at practice level is the creation of new knowledge where case presentations by students offer opportunities for the whole practice area to share in the new learning. The challenge is the required resources needed to keep the learning local and time for clinicians to attend; on the other hand, when attended by other professionals, especially senior staff, it reinforces the value of learning as a culture in the practice area.

Thinking about your Organisation

How would you introduce CLiP into your organisation?
How would you introduce CLiP to your practice area?
Which senior managers need to be involved in implementing CLiP?
How might this be managed?

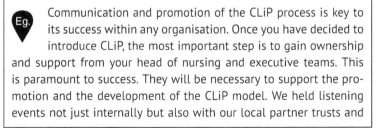

Communication and promotion of the CLiP process is key to its success within any organisation. Once you have decided to introduce CLiP, the most important step is to gain ownership and support from your head of nursing and executive teams. This is paramount to success. They will be necessary to support the promotion and the development of the CLiP model. We held listening events not just internally but also with our local partner trusts and community services, and working collaboratively with our hosting HEI. The development of posters and media promotion aided the process as did leaflet drops to ward areas.

It is key to gain voluntary buy-in from the wards you wish to use; this enables the ward managers to promote it within their own teams on a regular basis and embed the process early. The ward manager also shares this with patients and relatives so that they are also included in the development of the model within the area.

We held fortnightly steering group meetings which had representatives from the education team, wards, head of nursing, HEIs, and our local HEE offices. This enabled us to work through the logistics of the development of the project and set guidelines and design the teaching method we chose to train our wards in.

We had a designated CLiP lead within the organisations that supported the development of the process and coordinated the roll out. As a trust, we believe this is a vital role and one we still have today.

 Go to the companion website to see our CLiP journey and an example of a management structure to implement and support CLiP.

Collaboration at the student interface involves collaboration between coach and student, and student to student. The principle is shared learning through discovery, recognising and encouraging students to bring new learning to practice. Ford et al. (2016) from the supervisor perspective found that working with students was a motivator for supervisors to actively maintain and update their own knowledge.

At the time we were developing CLiP, there had been limited literature on collaborative learning between nursing students in the clinical environment. Subsequently, emerging evidence has supported our experience that peer learning improves the learning experience, enhancing confidence and self-efficacy (Tolsgard et al. 2016; Stenberg and Carlson 2015) with the emerging evaluative research on CLiP (see Chapter 6) endorsing this view. There have been some challenges; namely competition for supervisor time and non-compatible student dyads, where the dyads remained unchanged for the whole of the placement time (Stenberg and Carlson 2015; Nygren and Carlson 2017). In the CLiP model, student collaboration is team based involving three students at different levels in their training. Also, in the event a dyadic pairing cannot be avoided, then it is important that the pairing is not static for the whole placement but changes with different shifts as would happen in real-life practice. It is to be noted that some of the studies cited are based on simulated practice and not the clinical environment and thus do not consider the dynamics of social learning in a real-life situation and the influences of the wider clinical team on learning. Further, Tolsgard et al.'s (2016) review only focused on clinical skill development and not on the wider, complex professional skills acquired and developed in practice.

Real-Life Learning

The principle of real-life learning is that students learn to practice as a nurse right from the start. 'Learning to nurse' is a key theme of the report of the Willis Commission (2012: p. 32) which proposes that real-life care lies at the heart of patient-centred care and learning to be a nurse. Ford et al. (2016) suggest the most helpful form of supervising nurse is one who exposes their students to real-life situations, allowing the right balance between autonomy in care delivery and supported facilitation.

At an individual level, real-life learning involves students taking responsibility for total patient care, to be able to account for the care they plan and deliver commensurate with their level of practice. The allocation of patient(s) to student is collaborative and appropriate to the care setting, student status, competence, confidence, and learning objectives identified by the student. For example, a first-year first ward student will need to work very closely with their coach or mentor in their first week or two of placement, but might be able to take responsibility for the care of one patient by week two. Similarly, a third-year student might care for a group of patients or work with a more junior student, and a second-year student might be responsible for care of patients with more complex needs.

Our experience of student learning supports the view that students want independence as well as someone close at hand to offer continuous constructive feedback (Sandvik et al. 2014). In the CLiP model, students take the lead in care planning and discussions about care with the patient, their relatives, and the wider multidisciplinary team; they lead the handover of care to the next shift/practitioner, but always through direct or indirect supervision by the coach. However, it is recognised that there will be occasions when a more directive approach is required, such as in a crisis situations, low competence levels of practice, or failing students.

Real-life learning involves the need for students to work in a team structure that reflects the organisation of the ward/placement area. Being part of a team contributes to the student's sense of belonginess and feeling valued, an important prerequisite for learning (Courtney-Pratt et al. 2012). Thus, if patients are allocated to the registered nurse who will be the coach, then the patients will be divided between the students. However, if patients are allocated to a team consisting of a registered nurse and a healthcare assistant, then the work needs to be divided between the whole team and the healthcare assistant might be allocated to work with the first year delivering shared care, or be allocated to the third-year student who might delegate care. This is an important consideration taking into account the skill mix incorporated in healthcare delivery in the UK.

How Might you Create a Real-Life Learning Environment in your Practice Area?

How can it be organised, taking into account skill mix?
What might you need to do to protect student learning?

Here is an example of the experience of a community hospital

Specialism: Elderly rehabilitation, with sub-acute dependency patients
Beds: 24 beds
Staffing: 15 RNs, 15 HCAs. Staff on the ward work 12 and 7.5 hour shifts.
Student numbers: 10

Proactive and dynamic leadership, with good team involvement, enabled the implementation to run; relations with the university were strong and formal staff preparation was undertaken by the HEI

(Continued)

(Continued)

link lecturer, reinforced by more informal sessions with the ward manager. Good attendance was achieved at the on-site training of coaching the coaches. The ward initially assigned two learning bays for student allocation and one member of staff designated to coaching.

Prior to placement, students were provided with an introductory session to coaching. Additionally, the first two weeks of placement were dedicated to induction, whereby students orientated themselves to the practice area and patient group.

Initially, half the ward and one coach were reallocated to CLiP, but subsequently there has been a change in the ward's' staffing preventing the allocation of a coach to a bay. As a result of this, students now choose their own allocated patients, who are situated throughout the ward, based on learning opportunities, continuity of care, and student negotiated preference. The students" coach is allocated to lead a team containing the students but is not additionally responsible for the management of the ward.

Students have a resource room, dedicated folders for their daily learning logs, and are provided with an hour each shift for learning and the completion of the learning log, which is then checked by the coach. Feedback from the coach to the student's assessor is sometimes problematic, but the small, cohesive team manage assessment of practice completion in a timely fashion.

 Go to the companion website to see more examples.

Henderson et al. (2012) argue that it is not just the immediate coach–student relationship but also the interpersonal interactions that students have with the wider clinical team that shape their professional development. In the CLiP model, students are expected (under supervision) to liaise directly with the wider multidisciplinary team. Thus, for this to happen in a meaningful way, the whole practice area needs to commit to real-life learning at the practice level and this commitment and engagement has the potential to significantly enhance the culture of a practice area.

Real-life learning reflects the everyday running of the practice area, but this may create aspects of placements that are not necessarily student-focused. For example, students need to negotiate break cover between themselves and so may not be able to take the same breaks as their peers or supervisors. Further, students may not always have the continuity of working with the same coaches/mentors/fellow students, which have been described as important aspects of quality learning (Jokelainen et al. 2013, Courtney-Pratt et al. 2012).

Time to Teach and Time to Learn

This principle covers the organisation of student placement at an individual and practice level to create time to teach and time to learn. In our experience and as reflected in the literature, a main complaint from students on their placement experiences has been that mentors did not have time to teach students and students felt they were being used as an extra pair of hands (Hamshire et al. 2012). There is a view that the perceived 'business' of placement compromises learning opportunities and skill development and priority is often accorded to completing tasks (Stayt and Merrimen 2013; Courtney-Pratt et al. 2012). Our experience would support the view that the heavy workload of supervisors, the lack of acknowledgement of extra time needed to support and facilitate learning, compromises the quality of supervision (Clements et al. 2016) and suggests that the practice of care delivery is more valued than teaching and learning, which is often considered as secondary (Henderson and Eaton 2013). Thus, a vital aspect of the CLiP model is that the coach is freed up exclusively to supervise students and students are protected from the general business of ward practice, providing time to teach and time to learn. For students, the allocation of a limited number of patients to care for, the opportunity to negotiate the level of supervision required, the ability to access learning resources in the course of the day, and multiple opportunities for case discussion, all merge to provide a useful amount of time for learning.

The ability to apply the CLiP model in practice requires the support and commitment of the whole practice area. Henderson and Eaton (2013) claim that healthcare delivery is primarily focused on care provision with teaching and learning being a secondary activity when time permits – and there is a lack of understanding by management regarding the time taken to assist learners, discuss clinical situations, and provide feedback and that supervisors need protected time. They contend a task-orientated culture strongly prevails within the clinical learning environment. Thus, in the CLiP model at a practice level, student learning needs to be organised in a way that protects them from the general business of practice. This can be achieved whereby ward areas are designated 'student bays/student wings' and students are protected to learn and not drawn into the general ward/workplace culture where task performance and completion is the valued culture; instead, the organisation demonstrates its recognition and value of the importance of learning.

What Do you Think Are the Barriers that Prevent Supervisors from Having Time to Teach?

How could these be overcome?

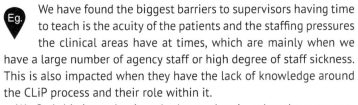

We have found the biggest barriers to supervisors having time to teach is the acuity of the patients and the staffing pressures the clinical areas have at times, which are mainly when we have a large number of agency staff or high degree of staff sickness. This is also impacted when they have the lack of knowledge around the CLiP process and their role within it.

We find this is predominantly due to the view that the extra students require extra work; whereas if you have staffing issues, the extra students can greatly help with delivery of care. At this point the education team would intervene to provide peer and education support to change the mindset and embed the foundations of CLiP within the teams and enable them to feel confident to step back and allow learner's to step up.

Go to the companion website to see how a coach made time for student learning: 'A day in the life of a coach'.

We found one of the challenges of CLiP is the level of intensity of supervision needed at the commencement of the student placement when the students are new to the practice area. There is a need for a higher level of direct supervision and observation in order to establish the baseline of a student's practice competence, this is particularly complex if all students start the placement at the same time. However, we also found that this lessened over time where CLiP was inculcated in the learning culture.

Stepping up and Stepping Back

Stepping up and stepping back reflects the coaching philosophy at the individual level whereby students 'step up' by taking more responsibility for their learning and delivery of care, and the coach 'steps back' allowing students to lead the care, playing a more facilitative role in their learning. Sandvik et al. (2014) found that students want an 'active approach to learning' where everything is not always explained, their thinking is critically challenged, and they are stimulated into enquiry. Ford et al. (2016) describe how students developed confidence and competence in clinical practice by being able to practise delivering hands-on care, allowing them to make and learn from their own mistakes: '… allow students to do their work without jumping in all the time' (Ford et al. 2016 : p. 100). An obvious caveat to this is for the supervisor to be able to intervene should the mistake cause harm in any way.

Think about Stepping up and Stepping Back

What might stop you giving a student full autonomy to practice? What does the NMC say about your responsibilities?

A lot of the time we found that it is the supervisor lack of confidence in their knowledge and ability and fear of giving away control of their care and it is a fallacy about giving away accountability because the student is accountable if they fail to work within the boundaries set. As long as supervisors prep students to do the care, and students are given the right information at the right time, the right support, coaching, and guidance, then the accountability then falls on the student if they go away and do something outside of those guidelines or scope of capability. It is the supervisor's confidence and capability

(Continued)

(Continued)

to be able to assess the students competence and that is where we will come in as the education support team to help embed the CLiP principles.

 Go to the companion website to see what students say about their hopes and experiences of practice.

The success of this principle is dependent on two main factors: first, a trusting and respectful relationship between coach and student, the responsibility of which predominantly lies with the coach. This relationship is based on a coaching philosophy of equality and collaboration, openness and honesty, unconditional positive regard, and a belief in the resourcefulness of the student (Rogers et al. 2012). Second is the ability and confidence of the coach to be able to accurately assess and document students' competence and the ability of the coach to match the student's competence and confidence with the right coaching style (NMC 2018 2.3); the coach needs to be able to assess whether the student has the confidence and competence to manage care delivery autonomously or, on the other end of the scale, needs close direct supervision to deliver care. In the CLiP model, we initially used Blanchard's situational leadership II model (Blanchard et al. 1985) as the theoretical framework to support this principle. However, we have now developed and adapted it to produce the 'framework to facilitate learning' which better reflects the student's learning journey from a nursing and midwifery perspective (see Chapter 7). Generally, students are expected to start their shift with pre-planned learning objectives identified in their learning logs which are completed on a daily basis, recording the learning achieved, and signed by the coach. The design of the learning log is based on and used to capture the evidence of competence that becomes evident through discussion or observation.

The notion of 'stepping back' not only allows students to learn by doing, but also facilitates the student to develop their thinking. It is a move away from the notion of mentor as expert, telling, explaining, and guiding; instead, using a questioning style to establish the student's knowledge base, identifying the theoretical basis of their practice, and helping students identify their own knowledge or practice gaps and consider creative solutions to care (NMC 2018 SSSA 2.6). Students in practice not only develop clinical skills but also need to develop critical thinking, the ability to use evidence judiciously, and to develop creative solutions to care. To seek advice, question and explore practice, students need a relationship that is safe and secure that enables them to feel included and valued and that helps motivate them (Henderson et al. 2012). According to Sandvik et al. (2014), the creation of a learning environment where students feel safe and secure to learn is a caring relationship that mirrors the nurse–patient caring relationship and is a 'prerequisite for learning and development'. This very much reflects the coach–student relationship advocated in the CLiP model, where all conversations are supported by coaching principles, and which is explored in detail in Part 2 of this book.

Feedback and Assessment

This principle of the CLiP model is focused at the individual level on the ability of the coach to assess competency, to be able to evidence and articulate how the competency is assessed, and feed back the performance to students. Further, the ability to assess, articulate, and evidence competence is vital in ensuring student and patient safety (NMC 2018 SSSA 2.4). Although it is generally recognised that competency encompasses three elements – knowledge, skills, and behaviour – the complexity of assessing these components individually or collectively in clinical practice remains a challenge (Zasadny and Bull 2015; Allen and Molloy 2017) and underpinning knowledge, despite being a key component of skill acquisition, is seldom discussed or assessed (Stayt and Merrimen 2013).

 Thinking about Student Competence

How confident are you in your ability to assess your student's competence? How do you do this?

What criteria do you use?

How do you document the evidence?

(Continued)

(Continued)

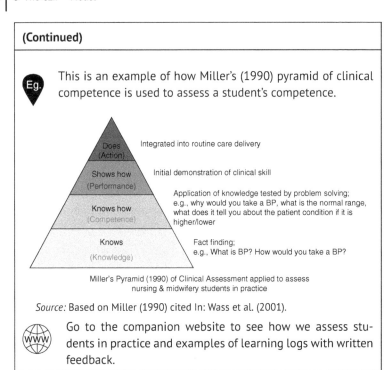

This is an example of how Miller's (1990) pyramid of clinical competence is used to assess a student's competence.

Integrated into routine care delivery

Initial demonstration of clinical skill

Application of knowledge tested by problem solving; e.g., why would you take a BP, what is the normal range, what does it tell you about the patient condition if it is higher/lower

Fact finding; e.g., What is BP? How would you take a BP?

Does (Action)

Shows how (Performance)

Knows how (Competence)

Knows (Knowledge)

Miller's Pyramid (1990) of Clinical Assessment applied to assess nursing & midwifery students in practice

Source: Based on Miller (1990) cited In: Wass et al. (2001).

Go to the companion website to see how we assess students in practice and examples of learning logs with written feedback.

There is a significant body of literature that identifies the vital role feedback plays in the learning and development of students (Jokelainen et al. 2013; Henderson and Eaton 2013; Sandvik et al. 2014). Sandvik et al. (2014) identify will and motivation as a prerequisite for learning and development, suggesting that students are generally internally motivated to learn but it is the quality of the feedback on their development and achievements that strengthens and drives this motivation. Further, they suggest that lack of feedback is mentally stressful as they struggle to make sense of how well they are doing, knowing where they stand, and whether things were done correctly or not. Ford et al. (2016) highlight understanding the assessment criteria as the most critical information needed by supervising nurses and claim there is a general lack of understanding of curriculum and assessment requirements.

In the CLiP model, it is expected that feedback is given in a contemporaneous way; thus, if a clinical skill was being supervised, then feedback would be given immediately after the procedure. During the course of the shift, it is expected that the coach and team reconvene periodically to review how the work is progressing and feedback is given during these occasions – and finally feedback is given individually at the end of each shift/day when completing the learning log. The learning log is a mechanism that enables a 'coaching conversation' to be conducted within the context of the student's learning journey; i.e., establishing the level of competency and support requirements of the student in relation to their learning objectives/outcomes. The learning logs should be filled out daily, kept in the practice area, and should be cross-referenced to any practice assessment document. We would advocate that the use of daily learning logs is vital with the new standards for student supervision and assessment (NMC 2018).

Look Back at the Last Couple of Feedback Sessions you Have Had with Students

When did you give the feedback?
How often did you do this?
What did you say/write?
How do you think the student might use the feedback you gave to improve their performance/do better next time?

Here is an example of a daily learning log with written feedback.

Collaborative Learning in Practice Learning Log			
Name of Student: 2nd yr. Adult community placement Module 3 Name of coach: Date:			
Assessment of competency: 1 = Knows 2 = Knows how 3 = Shows how 4 = Does	Stages of Competency: S1 = low competency S2 = low/some competence S3 = mod/high competence S4 = High competence	Required coaching style: D1 = Directive D2 = Coaching D3 = Support D4 = Delegating	Goal Achieved

(Continued)

(Continued)

Overview of Learning Outcome:
Learning outcome 4 - Care of patient with leg ulcer

Learning objectives/ goals for the day (student to fill in)	Expectation from coach (student to fill in)	Assessment of competency (coach to fill in)	Coach signature

• Meet Mrs. A
• Familiarise myself with patient medical and social history
  o Understand the causes of leg ulcers
• What does a home visit involve
• Care of leg ulcer
  o How is aseptic technique adapted in the community?
  o Access wound
  o Identify treatment/ dressing options
	Help with accessing electronic notes
	
	Demonstrate the preparation and delivery of wound dressing
		Used 'Hello my name is'
		Has observed how to access patient notes
		
		Has observed where to retrieve dressings from health centre
		
		Not clear about leg ulcer assessment
		
		Observed clean technique for wound dressing
			AB

Student self-reflection	Coach feedback
	Feedback on professional behaviour and performance, reassess competency in relation to the days agreed L/O discuss unexpected achievements Gained patient consent competently Was very respectful in patient's own home, recognised professional boundaries *Feedforward any areas in need of development, any agreed actions or suggestions for future learning* 1. Needs to understand the A&P of wound healing in order to assess leg ulcers 2. Review causes of leg ulcers 3. Next time will undertake wound dressing under supervision 4. Consider the wider implications in caring for a person with wounds, e.g. social conditions, diet, infection control

Student signature:

Coach signature:

Go to the webpage to hear what students say about the feedback they receive and to see further examples of learning logs.

Allen and Molloy (2017) in their study of the use of a daily feedback tool found it useful in overcoming barriers such as frequency and style of feedback. They found that effective feedback enhanced trust in the student–supervisor relationship, which in turn enabled students to be proactive in seeking feedback.

The model presented in this chapter has explained the theoretical underpinnings that support the development of the CLiP model of practice education. Subsequent to its development, there have been a number of research studies undertaken of this model and they are presented in Chapter 6.

References

Allen, L. and Molloy, E. (2017). The influence of a preceptor-student 'daily feedback tool' on clinical feedback practices in nursing education: a qualitative study. *Nurse Education Today* 49: 57–62.

Blanchard, K., Zigarmi, P., and Zigarmi, D. (1985). *Leadership and the One Minute Manager: Increasing Effectiveness through Situational Leadership.* New York: Morrow.

Clements, A., Kinman, G., Leggetter, S. et al. (2016). Exploring commitment, professional identity, and support for student nurses. *Nurse Education in Practice* 16: 20–26.

Courtney-Pratt, H., FitzGerald, M., Ford, K. et al. (2012). Quality clinical placements for undergraduate nursing students: a cross-sectional survey of undergraduates and supervising nurses. *Journal of Advanced Nursing* 68 (6): 1380–1390.

Duffy, K. (2003). Failing students: a qualitative study of factors that influence the decisions regarding the assessment of students' competence in practice. Available online at: http://science.ulster.ac.uk/nursing/mentorship/docs/nursing/oct11/failingstudents.pdf (accessed 15 June 2020).

Ford, K., Courtney-Pratt, H., Marlow, A. et al. (2016). Quality clinical placements: the perspectives of undergraduate nursing students and their supervising nurses. *Nurse Education Today* 37: 97–102.

Hamshire, C., Willgoss, T., and Wibberler, C. (2012). 'The placement was probably the tipping point'. The narratives of recently discontinued students. *Nurse Education in Practice* 12 (4): 182–186.

Henderson, A. and Eaton, E. (2013). Assisting nurses to facilitate student and new graduate learning in practice settings: what 'support' do nurses at the bedside need? *Nurse Education in Practice* 13 (3): 197–201.

Henderson, A., Cooke, M., Creedy, D., and Walker, R. (2012). Nursing students' perceptions of learning in practice environments: a review. *Nurse Education Today* 32 (3): 299–302.

Jokelainen, M., Turunen, H., Tossavainen, J.D., and Coco, K. (2011). A systematic review of mentoring nursing students in linical placements. *Journal of Clinical Nursing* 20 (19–20): 2854–2867.

Jokelainen, M., Jamookeeah, D., Tossavainen, K., and Turunen, H. (2013). Finnish and British mentors' conceptions of facilitating nursing students' placement learning and professional development. *Nurse Education in Practice* 13 (1): 61–67.

Kelton, M. (2014). Clinical coaching – an innovative role to improve marginal nursing students' clinical practice. *Nurse Education in Practice* 14 (6): 709–713.

Levett-Jones, T. and Lathlean, J. (2008). Belonginess: a prerequisite for nursing students' clinical learning. *Nurse Education in Practice* 8: 103–111.

Miller, G.E. (1990). The assessment of clinical skills/competence/performance. *Academic Medicine* 65: S63–S67.

Nursing and Midwifery Council (NMC) (2008). *Standards to Support Learning and Assessment in Practice*. London: NMC.

Nursing and Midwifery Council (NMC) (2018). Standards for student supervision and assessment. www.nmc.org.uk/standards-for-education-and-training/standards-for-student-supervision-and-assessment (accessed 2 December 2020).

Nygren, F. and Carlson, E. (2017). Preceptors' conceptions of a peer learning model: a phenomenographic study. *Nurse Education Today* 49: 12–16.

Rogers, J., Gilbert, A., and Whittleworth, K. (2012). *Manager as Coach, the New Way to Get Results*. Maidenhead: McGraw-Hill.

Sandvik, A., Eriksson, K., and Hilli, Y. (2014). Becoming a caring nurse – a Nordic study on students' learning and development in clinical education. *Nurse Education in Practice* 14 (3): 286–292.

Stayt, L. and Merrimen, C. (2013). A descriptive survey investigating pre-registration student nurses' perceptions of clinical skill development in clinical placements. *Nurse Education Today* 33: 425–430.

Stenberg, M. and Carlson, E. (2015). Swedish student nurses' perception of peer learning as an educational moel during clinical practice in a hospital setting – an evaluation study. *BMC Nursing* 14: 48. https://bmcnurs.biomedcentral.com/articles/10.1186/s12912-015-0098-2.

Tolsgard, M., Kulasegaram, K., and Ringsted, C. (2016). Collaborative learning of clinical skills in health professions education: the why, how, when and for whom. *Medical Education* 50 (1): 69–78.

Wass, V., Van der Vleuten, C., Shatzer, J. and Jones, R. (2001). Assessment of clinical competence. *The Lancet* 357: 945–949.

Willis Commission (2012). *Quality with Compassion: The Future of Nursing Education*. London: RCN.

Zasadny, M. and Bull, R. (2015). Assessing competence in undergraduate nursing students: the amalgamated students assessment in practice model. *Nurse Education in Practice* 15 (2): 126–133.

4

System-Wide Approaches to CLiP™

4.1

The South West CLiP™ Community Cluster Project
Jane Bunce

Background and Drivers

During 2017/18 it became evident to Health Education England South West (HEE-SW) and others, through the Devon, Cornwall, and Isles of Scilly Quality Surveillance Group, that care homes and nursing beds were closing, in part due to the inability to recruit qualified nurses to these settings. It was recognised that this not only impacts on patients being cared for closer to home, but on the wider NHS system, in terms of discharging patients from the acute care setting to the community. The Collaborative Learning in Practice (CLiP™) Community Cluster (CCC) Project was instigated to explore whether a CLiP model of learning had the potential to address this situation by raising the quality of placements in the community and thus ultimately encouraging recruitment of adult nurses (Health Education England 2017a,b) to the community.

Why CLiP?

CLiP moves away from the traditional one-to-one mentorship model in favour of a coaching approach where students work in groups to lead the care for an allocated number of patients. Students support and learn from each other whilst being overseen by any registered professional. CLiP is potentially beneficial in the above circumstances because it enables a higher number of students to be placed in these settings whilst also reducing the burden on individual mentors (Clarke et al. 2018). The quality of the learning environment can increase by students becoming part of a truly multiprofessional team, allowing staff time to teach and students to learn, whilst better preparing them for practice (Lobo 2016). In the acute setting, CLiP has been widely piloted across the United Kingdom; however, there was limited experience within the community at the time of the CLiP CCC project.

Project Overview

The project was led by HEE-SW in collaboration with the Devon, Cornwall, and Somerset Training Hubs and the University of Plymouth, thus taking a systems leadership approach to benefit learners and ultimately the patient. Limited research had been conducted with CliP; therefore, in addition to the project budget, a sum of money was identified to fund research led by Plymouth University and HEE-SW. The Project Manager also led a trip to Amsterdam, where CLiP originated as the real-life learning ward (Lobo et al. 2014; Health Education England 2017a,b). The project commenced in April 2018 and concluded on 2 April 2019.

How Was CLiP Implemented in the Pilot Sites?

During an initial planning workshop, it became clear that project stakeholders wanted to pilot CLiP in a variety of community settings. Therefore, project placements involved in the pilot included primary care, hospices, and nursing homes. Placements used had previously taken one to three students at a time, while the nursing homes had not offered placements previously. The placement period ran with second- and third-year students between October and December 2018. In addition to increasing student capacity, the aim was to offer an enhanced learning experience for students using the CliP model. Table 4.1.1 outlines the pilot sites and the student placement numbers, which represent a 300% increase in students.

A Healthcare Practice Placement Development Lead (PPDL) from the university provided the preparation activity prior to placements. This included a briefing for students and preparation sessions for staff, which introduced them to the CLiP model and how this might work in

Table 4.1.1   Placement capacity: 2018 CLiP CC Pilot.

	Total capacity	2nd yr	3rd yr
Plymouth			
Hospice	6	4	2
GP surgery	6	3	3
Nursing home	6	3	3
Somerset			
Care home	4	2	2
Hospice	6	3	3
GP surgery	5	3	2
Cornwall			
Nursing home[a]	3	2	1

a) Placements were pulled prior to completion due to patient safety issues reported by students.

practice. When the pilot commenced, the students received a further briefing on how things would work and weekly reflection sessions were facilitated. The PPDL attended site visits and was contactable via email and telephone throughout the placement period.

The project culminated in a Celebrating Collaborative Learning Conference in Exeter in May 2019. The conference brought together a range of attendees from across the UK and Amsterdam to share current research and good practice in collaborative learning.

What Worked Well in the Pilot?

- Increased capacity achieved.
- Local, regional, and international links established; and sharing of good practice.
- Enhanced patient care in some areas: e.g., in one GP practice dedicated student-led BP clinics took place; increased appointment time (756 patients).

- Social prescribing through widening access to a gardening club, facilitated by students through development of a social media site/campaign.
- Students in GP were trained in venepuncture and able to utilise these skills in practice.
- Preparation for new NMC standards – exposure to coaching model – staff and students.
- Enhanced exposure to end of life and palliative care.
- Students benefitted from learning together and supporting each other.
- Real-life problem-solving experience.
- Recruitment into primary care – permanent and bank staff.

At the time of writing, a piece of research is being conducted to determine whether patient care has improved as a result of CLiP.

What Were the Main Challenges?

- Preparation is key for staff and it should be recognised that students do not necessarily fully understand CLiP until they have started to operationalise the model.
- Putting coaching models into practice was more challenging for some than others.
- Some staff felt uncomfortable standing back and letting students lead patient care.
- Managing students in larger groups was a challenge for some due to squabbling and unexpected power struggles.
- Some areas felt that there were too many students on placement.

What Did We Decide we Would Do Differently Following the Pilot?

- Reduce the number of students to an agreed number for community CLiP placements.
- Enhance student preparation around how CLiP works, roles, and responsibilities and expectations.
- Plan any training such as phlebotomy to take place in first week.

- Students now receive preparation for peer coaching through all three years of study and CLiP will be mirrored in clinical skills training.
- Include planned scheduled learning sessions for students – could be part of weekly reflection events.
- Enhance staff preparation around coaching for student nurse clinical practice.
- Enhance staff preparation and support for managing student group dynamics.

References

Clarke, D., Williamson, G.R., and Kane, A. (2018). *Could Students' Experiences of Clinical Placements Be Enhanced by Implementing a Collaborative Learning in Practice (CLiP) Model?* Nurse Education in Practice: Elsevier.

Health Education England (2017a). Case study: implementing collaborative learning in practice – a new way of learning for nursing students. Workforce Information Network.

Health Education England (2017b). Reducing pre-registration attrition and improving recruitment report. https://www.hee.nhs.uk/our-work/reducing-pre-registration-attrition-improving-retention (accessed 12 January 2020).

Lobo, C. (2016). Collaborative Learning in Practice (CLiP): A systematic approach to practice education (unpublished manuscript).

Lobo, C., Arthur, A., and Lattimer, V. (2014). *Collaborative Learning in Practice (CLiP) for Pre-Registration Nursing Students.* Health Education England University of East Anglia.

4.2

Lancashire Teaching Hospitals NHS Foundation Trust Implementation of the CLiP™ Model of Supervision
Jonty Kenward

Background and Drivers

Lancashire Teaching Hospitals recognised the need to increase placement capacity in line with the national drive upon the removal of both the bursary and the HEI student cap. It was deemed appropriate to implement the CLiP model here at Lancashire Teaching Hospitals, which is one of the largest and highest performing trusts in the country. We provide district general hospital services to 370 000 people in Preston and Chorley, and specialist care to 1.5 million people across Lancashire and South Cumbria. The project fulfils the ethos of the Health Education North West Strategic Plan (2015/16), Francis (2013), Keogh (2013), Willis Commission (2012), Berwick (2013), and the Cavendish (2013) Reports. These highlight the need to develop the workforce fit for the purpose of meeting the increasing need for high-quality healthcare, delivered by professionals who are able to meet this demand with relevant expertise and knowledge. This includes recruiting more individuals onto healthcare courses, reducing attrition, and increasing the numbers of healthcare learners achieving their qualification. The increasing number of nursing students is placing great demand upon placement capacity. Therefore, it was envisaged that the CLiP project would ease the pressure, by increasing placement capacity. The current model of student allocation to placement is inconsistent, as it is reliant on the educational audit process, which sets the limits to each area dependent on multiple factors.

Key Aims

We aimed to provide an enhanced and different placement experience for mentors and students.

1. To demonstrate to the NW how placement capacity could be increased.
2. To promote a quality learning environment.
3. To enable the learners to be functioning members of a multidisciplinary team (MDT).
4. To build confidence and competence within our learners.
5. To develop our current and future workforce, enabling interprofessional learning.

We aimed to improve student placement satisfaction with regards to student feedback from several reporting mechanisms. Students were voicing concerns that in some areas placements were not expecting them, that mentors were too busy to teach, and there were generally insufficient educational resources and staffing in practice to support them.

It was proposed that the project would play an important role in the retention of students by helping to eliminate these concerns. The CLiP approach removes the requirement for learners to work directly with their mentors on a one-to-one basis. This is mainly due to coaching that is provided by all levels of staff and working on a team approach to support. However, learners are still overseen by overarching qualified mentors who maintain responsibility for care delivery. Mentors vocalise that CLiP enables them to fulfil their role, by changing the ethos from instruction to coaching, questioning, and stepping back to allow the students to step forward and become critical thinkers. We aim to produce a future workforce that is confident and competent upon completion of their courses, which in turn impacts on the care delivered to our patients and their families.

Implementation

We initially requested volunteer ward areas; this was so we had ward-level ownership for the implementation of the project. Expressions of interest were requested following a visit from the placement lead at

UEA who presented their findings within the work they had undertaken there. We felt that if the ward managers volunteered, they would be able to support and promote the process within their teams. Our two volunteer wards were Male Neurosurgical and Burns and Plastics. We launched a steering group 12 months prior to the launch on the ward areas in September 2015. The membership consisted of placement development managers, head of placement support team at LTHTr, head of nursing, a senior lecturer from both main HEI partners, UCLAN and Bolton, a student quality ambassador, two voluntary ward managers, and a member of the organisational development team who would be involved in the development and delivery of the coaching sessions. In this meeting, terms of reference were designed and future meeting dates were set up to deliver the outcomes of the project.

In October 2015, an application to Health Education England NW was submitted to support the project moving forward. This was agreed in March 2016, which allowed for consultancy fees, advertising materials, payments to staff attending coaching sessions, and support of the project in the two pilot CLiP areas.

In February 2016, the first coaching session commenced and all advertising materials were designed and ordered. The pilot was also introduced at a retention event hosted by HEENW.

Advertising commenced in March 2016, posters were displayed in the pilot areas – 'CLiP is coming' – and leaflets given to staff, patients, and students. Ward managers discussed it with all staff at daily board meetings and gave information at the front line. The placement support team and PEFs conducted pre project sessions which gave insight into the project and how it would impact the teams.

Questionnaires were circulated to staff, students, and patients to give a benchmark for satisfaction of service delivery. April 2016 saw the cascade of coaching workshops with 26 staff from both pilot areas attending for several two-hours sessions. Students were prepared by lecturers from both the university partners.

The project commenced on 31 May 2016 in both pilot areas. Our original student figures on the two wards were 8 and 10 and we increased them both to 20 students per placement, which was a total of 122% in just two areas. The ward was then separated into learning bays. A coach would facilitate the learning of a minimum of three students, dependent on the level of experience and year group. They would coach the learners to undertake holistic care of a group of patients, developing their essential skills, documentation, ward rounds, and handovers to the next shift. The coaches were overseen and kept in contact with over-arching mentors who maintained responsibility, completed the student's documentation, and provided support where required.

Students were requested to complete learning logs as a reflective account of activity in relation to their competencies. These would be signed and commented on by the coaches each day and held as evidence for their named mentors in relation to the completion of their student documentation.

The project culminated in the CLiP conference held at the Health Academy in September 2016, where we shared our success and journey with delegates from across the region.

What Worked Well on Implementation

- Increased capacity achieved.
- Enhanced patient care, shown in ward harm-free care figures.
- Student peer support was recognised as invaluable.
- Increased sense of MDT/inter-professional learning.
- Able to demonstrate key learning to North West regional partners.
- Increased mentor and student satisfaction.
- Increased confidence levels at an early stage.
- Local, regional, and international links.
- Preparation for the NMC standard changes.
- Increased retention of future workforce.

What Were the Main Challenges?

- The logistics of implementing the project and level of support required on opening up a CLiP area.
- Obtaining financial support to enable coaching sessions to take place.
- Staff attendance at the cascade coaching sessions.
- Full attendance at the steering group.
- Managing expectations of all parties.
- Managing anxiety levels.
- Staff felt uncomfortable when being asked to step back; they queried levels of accountability.

- Duty rosters for larger groups of learners.
- Too many learners.
- Implementation of learning logs.

It is important to be organised, have contingency plans, and try to keep to the proposed timeline. This is not a project that can be rushed through as it is a very labour-intensive process, which needs a lot of input by all staff involved.

Top Tips

- Take time to implement – at least three months per ward.
- Induction for learners held in house prior to placements.
- Continued named CLiP lead to support the process in the areas.
- Continuity and consistency of information given.
- Manage student off duty closely.
- Introduction of student diary to reflect the learning journey.
- Be open to change and recognise how to adapt in different areas.
- Utilise all levels of staff and recognise capability amongst teams.
- Share best practice and build key relationships to support the role.

References

Berwick, D. (2013). *A Promise to Learn – A Commitment to Act: Improving the Safety of Patients in England*. London: Department of Health.

Cavendish, C. (2013). *An Independent Enquiry into Healthcare Assistants and Support Workers in the NHS and Social Care Setting*. London: Department of Health and Social Care.

Francis, R. (2013). *Report of the Mid Staffordshire NHS Foundation Trust Public Inquiry*. London: The Stationery Office.

Health Education North West - Workforce Planning Round (2015/16). http://www.ewin.nhs.uk/tools_and_resources/health-education-north-west-workforce-planning-round-2015-2016 (accessed 2 December 2020).

Keogh, B. (2013). *Review into the Quality of Care and Treatment Provided by 14 Hospital Trusts in England: Overview Report*. London: NHS England.

Willis Commission (2012). *Quality with Compassion: The Future of Nursing Education*. London: RCN.

4.3

James Paget University NHS Foundation Trust Implementing the CLiP™ Model in Maternity Care

Kenda Crozier, Jodie Yerrell and Kirsty Tweedie

Introduction

The plan for implementation in maternity was devised and directed by the clinical educator who led training in the trial ward (Tweedie et al. 2019). The communication and messaging about the project was strong and consistent and identified the strong coalition of partners and commitment to the new way of supporting learning environments.

How Was CLiP Implemented?

Collaborative working between the UEA and the James Paget University NHS Foundation Trust led by the midwifery clinical educator and including the head of midwifery, lead midwife for education, and link lecturer from the university, with support from the course director, ward manager, midwives, and clinical educators from nursing.

This way of working required a model of transformational change to underpin the development and implementation and leadership skills, including engaging the team, sharing the vision, and evaluating information (NHS Leadership Academy skills 2013). Change is rarely a straightforward process from beginning to end, and for this transition there were some aspects that we will detail in order to provide learning for others considering embarking on the journey. The change can be explained using Kotter's eight-step model (Kotter 2012, 1996).

1. *Establishing a sense of urgency.*

   Primarily, the sense of urgency was driven by the desire to create a more equitable and student-led learning environment where the students took an active role in the identification and achievement of their own learning objectives. As this was being developed, the sense of urgency was further underpinned by an impetus to develop and sustain a model to increase capacity in maternity to enable the growth of student numbers. The recognition by the head of midwifery that there was a need to attract more students was driven by a need to develop the workforce and innovative service.

2. *Creating and maintaining guiding coalition.*

   The strong coalition was created by partnership working across nursing and midwifery clinical education, led in the Trust by the education lead for the CLiP model being active across all areas. The university supported initiatives to improve practice in service and education. The working relationship between the link lecturer and the clinical educator were important in providing the training in coaching. A broader model of coaching was also supported within the Trust as part of their leadership development programme. So, in short, buy-in from all parties to the model created a strength of purpose.

3. *Developing a change vision.*

   The vision was clear and was supported by the fact that success within nursing was being seen through positive evaluation by students and staff who were involved in coaching (Hill et al. 2020; Hill et al. 2015). Workshops were provided to train staff in both the model and coaching skills with educators, role-modelling coaching conversations. It was important to allay concerns about coaching as a new skill. Midwives already use many of the skills of coaching in their clinical practice. Consider the way midwives support women to make decisions about place of birth or pain relief: much of this involves enabling women to ask questions and to think through the options and then for women to come to informed decisions. The training also drew on the skills already used within the mentorship model (NMC 2008) that was at that time a routine part of midwifery education. Most midwives were used to taking a step back to enable student midwives to provide support and care for women. The learning environment was one of supporting development of a midwifery skills set to enable students to gain proficiency from a very early stage of their education programmes. Coaches were reassured that as with the existing model, students would be expected to step up to demonstrate their skills and knowledge but could also step back in situations where they were unsure. In situations where safety was an issue, coaches were encouraged to use direction as appropriate. The relationship of equality between coach and student was sometimes a difficult concept, as midwives who regard themselves as 'expert' could find it challenging not to control situations. They were encouraged in the training to consider scenarios when this could happen and alternative approaches where they could use their skills as coaches.

4. *Communicating the vision for buy-in.*
   Student projects were showcased within the trust in a celebratory way which enabled students and their coaches to feel valued. The multidisciplinary attendance at events where students shared their learning also helped to spread the vision across disciplinary boundaries. In addition to this, these shared learning opportunities led to further involvement in other projects for students where a common interest and learning was noted, such as student inclusion in ongoing service development and change initiatives developed within the Trust.

5. *Empowering broad-based action.*
   Undoubtably the support from leadership within the ward and from the head of midwifery enabled barriers to be broken down. Staff were provided with training time to attend sessions to help them understand the model and the clinical educator was on hand to support students and staff and to maintain clear messages about expectations of the model. The CLiP documentation of learning logs was adapted to fit the way in which midwives support student learning outcomes and the grading of practice element to ensure that students had a means to evidence their learning against the learning outcomes for their placements.

6. *Generating short-term wins.*
   Students taking responsibility for identifying their own learning needs is a fundamental element of the coaching process and exercises were created to enable the staff to consider and construct conversations using effective styles of questioning and listening. One aspect which is key to successful coaching is enabling students to develop solution-focused responses to situations which they may find difficult.

Coaches worked through role-play to learn how this could be done. The completion of learning logs and coaching forms, which formed part of the CLiP model, were also important in training to ensure that new paperwork would not be a hindrance to success of the trial.

The wholesale approach to supporting students across different year groups would mean a change in the entire placement circuit, affecting students on all programme years in all trusts partnered with the university, and it was clear that this could not be a quick process. Therefore, we decided on a quick win approach that would support the existing placement plan to trial the model before making changes to placements that would increase student numbers. This worked because staff gained confidence in the new ways of working before we moved forward with changes that increased numbers and introduced extra students with different levels of outcome requirements.

7. *Never letting up.*

Once we established the model, students themselves acted as champions and we were able to make placement circuit changes that ensured all three year groups were placed in the ward at the same time and provided with peer support. The students developed their coaching skills and the model developed in strength. This provided opportunities for senior students to coach not only their peer group, but also to support learning from students in years one and two of their programmes. The learners valued viewing each other's development and took pride in supporting each other.

8. *Incorporating changes into culture.*

This is probably one of the most significant aspects in the change process. It assumes that any change can be embedded in a static format. However, the NHS is ever-evolving and each organisation within it is dynamic. The challenge was not to create a process that would be static, but to enable the evolution of coaching to be flexible and sustainable so that it could respond to change. The selection of placement area was deliberate in that it most closely mirrored some of the nursing environments where CLiP had been successful. Once it was embedded, we needed to ensure that it was maintained and that the change could grow across other maternity areas, such as community and most importantly birthing settings. We have encountered changes including staff rotation, meaning that staff with coaching skills move to other areas. This is both a negative, in that the experience is lost from the original area, but also a positive in that it helps to create the momentum for change in another area. This aspect of cultural change is often the sticking point for transformation.

Timeline

The timeline to implementation was carefully thought through and agreed with all parties to meet a deadline for students arriving on the ward for the first placement of the academic year in October. You can see that this process effectively – and appropriately for maternity – took around nine months.

Top Tips

The original cohort of students has now qualified and champion coaching, the clinical educator who drove the implementation of CLiP has moved on, and many of the ward team have rotated. So, maintaining the learning culture must be planned carefully with regular reviews to ensure that when a new clinical educator comes on board, training and support is provided within the coalition to maintain quality.

- Preparing staff in the learning environment is one of the most important factors for success.
- Clinical education staff should be prepared to role-model the coaching and show confidence in the model. They need education and preparation to create and maintain learning cultures.
- Lasting change takes work; be wary of declaring success too early in the game.
- Any changes to placement rotation or student allocation, including increasing or decreasing student numbers, must consider the impact on the learning environment and the workability of the model.
- Prepare all students entering the learning environment, so they understand their role in learning.
- The coalition needs to be strong at the beginning and must be maintained and nurtured.
- Succession planning is vital. Clinical staff move on and clinical educators develop their careers in other directions.

References

Hill, R., Woodward, M., and Arthur, A. (2015). *Collaborative Learning in Practice (CLiP): Evaluation Report.* East Anglia: HEE East of England and University of East Anglia.

Hill, R., Woodward, M., and Arthur, A. (2020). Collaborative learning in practice (CLiP): evaluation of a new approach to clinical learning. *Nurse Education in Practice* 85 (2020): 104295.

Kotter, J.P. (1996). *Leading Change.* Cambridge, MA: Harvard Business School Press.

Kotter, J.P. (2012). Accelerate. *Harvard Business Review* 90 (November 2012): 44–58.

NHS Leadership Academy (2013). Healthcare Leadership Model. The nice dimensions of leadership behaviour. Leeds: NHS Leadership Academy.

NMC (2008). *Standards to Support Learning and Assessment in Practice*, 2008. London: NMC.

Tweedie, K., Yerrell, J., and Crozier, K. (2019). Collaborative coaching and learning in midwifery clinical placements. *British Journal of Midwifery* 27 (5): 324–329.

5

Coaching Theory and Models
Rachel Paul

One of the main differences between CLiP™ and the more traditional approaches to nurse and midwifery practice education has been the underlying philosophy on teaching and learning in practice. Historically, a strong didactic teaching approach has been used in practice learning for nursing and midwifery students, whereas CLiP is underpinned by a coaching philosophy where we are looking to apply coaching approaches to facilitate teaching and learning.

From our perspective there are some clear distinctions between coaching and teaching that we need to highlight. For us, teaching is a 'telling' activity – at a very basic level, teaching is instructing an individual on how to carry out a task and explaining what the reason is for carrying out that task. The taught individual is then expected to carry out the task they have been trained in. Coaching, on the other hand, assumes that the individual knows how to carry out the task but may or may not have already done so. Coaching is focused on what the student wants to do, improve, or resolve for themselves, without being told what to do; being encouraged to look for answers inside themselves and act on what they perceive is required. It follows then that advice giving is not necessarily required to develop a student's motivation and sense of resourcefulness. Rogers (2012: p. 51) stated 'You insist, I resist'. The more we, as educators, tell our students what to do, without giving them a chance to think and work out for themselves what they feel is needed, the more we treat them as children. This may then result in disempowering them from being the confident learners they need to be in order to learn from their mistakes and build resilience to grow into their profession.

Collaborative Learning in Practice: Coaching to Support Student Learners in Healthcare, First Edition. Charlene Lobo, Rachel Paul, and Kenda Crozier.
© 2021 John Wiley & Sons Ltd. Published 2021 by John Wiley & Sons Ltd.
Companion website: www.wiley.com/go/lobo/collaborativelearninginpractice

There are some key coaching skills and approaches that can support teaching. The core skills of questioning and listening, together with rapport building and feedback, can be used to create even more powerful and confidence-building opportunities. In this chapter we look at specific examples of doing just this.

It's worth remembering that there is always the option to mentor, and that where you have a trainee or student with little or no experience, mentoring may be the best option. Mentoring uses the same core skills of coaching – building rapport, questioning, and reflective listening. As part of the initial contracting process it is important to distinguish what you are offering your student.

The theory that underpins coaching is taken from that of educational development and adult learning (Kolb, 1984) as well as many psychological sources. Many coaching authors have noted that coaching theory is still growing and emerging. The main point to note is that when using coaching to develop professionals, the theories outlined here provide a taster of the ideas, frameworks, and tools for us to use so that we can be even more useful to those we support – either as a coach or as a facilitator of learning. Part 2 gives you the opportunity to look at how these coaching theories can be put into practice as well as hints and tips on how to do this.

Coaching Theory

There are lots of different theories that we could have included in this chapter but we are looking at just nine. Please don't let that put you off looking at others; for a comprehensive guide, look at Wildflower and Brennan (2011) The *Handbook of Knowledge-based Coaching* for further theoretical insight that comes with excellent hints for applying the theory. Before looking at the theory, it is important to familiarise ourselves with Rogers (2012: p. 7) (adapted to this context) six foundation principles of coaching, these have certainly supported my practice and many that have studied coaching.

The first principle is that the student is resourceful. Drawing on the ideas of adult learning and andragogy (Knowles in Wildflower and Brennan 2011: p. 74), the belief that students come into healthcare, midwifery, and nursing with experience and skills to resolve problems for themselves. After relevant training, the supervisor is able to coach the student to use their knowledge and experience base in practice, resisting the temptation to give information and advice. Although sometimes guidance is requested, and needed, the more advice giving that happens, the less likely it is that the student will develop confidence in themselves.

The second principle is that the coach's role is to develop the student's resourcefulness through skilful questioning, challenge and support. Coaching is not just a 'cosy' chat where the supervisor gives advice, but a space where issues or problems can be dealt with openly, and where the relationship between supervisor and student has clear boundaries and ground rules to create the environment of safety required for the student to reveal their need for support to overcome any learning challenges or barriers. Students that have different styles of learning need to be able to trust their supervisor to feel able to reveal what learning needs they have and work collaboratively with them.

The third principle, Rogers (2012: p. 8) reminds us, is that coaching addresses the whole person – their past, present, and future; work and private lives. The past potentially influences each of us in different ways and it is from our past that we can learn. We sometimes pretend we are two different people, one at work and one outside work. In fact, we are one person and what happens in one part of our life impacts on other areas.

The fourth principle of coaching is that the student sets the agenda. This might be seen to be problematic if the supervisor is used to a telling or didactic style of working. However, as soon as the supervisor begins to be learner led, the benefits of student-led solutions – buy-in to action planning, development of practice, and learning – become transparent.

The fifth principle builds on the notion communicated in the fourth of democracy; principle five is that the supervisor and student are equals. At the end of this chapter we look in more depth at transactional analysis and the inevitable presence of ego in interactions, but let's just keep in mind now the benefits of an equal adult to adult relationship and all that entails.

The sixth and final principle that Rogers (2012: p. 9) offers us is that coaching is about change and action. There must be lots of triggers of change in student worlds of learning and work. Coaching is about the resolution of those changes and working out ways of responding to change that is effective for all concerned. Building confidence and self-awareness is often a crucial outcome of coaching, leaving individuals more resourceful to cope with changes.

The Psychodynamic Coaching Approach

Lee in Cox, Bachkirova and Clutterbuck (2014: p. 22) argued there are four assumptions underpinning the psychodynamic approach, which has its roots in Freud (1922), Jung (1956), Kline (2015), and Siegel (2010).

Assumption One: Making Conscious What is Unconscious

We are often conscious of our behaviour, appearance, and even our language. However, we may not be so conscious of the beliefs, values, thoughts, feelings, habits, and assumptions that drive our behaviours. By identifying the personal drivers in our lives, we may increase our motivation to achieve our potential.

- The act of coaching involves the coachee talking – the coach actively encourages this through open and probing questioning which when combined with reflective listening helps the coachee to re-examine their experiences, reflect on their feelings, actions, and the thoughts stored in their unconscious.
- Verbalising what is going on in your head and your heart gives the coachee a chance to listen to themself as well as be heard by another person.
- Self-awareness can be a direct result of coaching – realisation of your contribution to a situation, both negative and positive, can be excellent for learning how to resolve issues.
- The act of making explicit what is implicit is comparable to researching ourselves and tapping into those hidden or unconscious values and beliefs that can propel us forward with solutions to act or hold ourselves back with self-limiting beliefs.

Assumption Two: Creating a Safe Space with Clear Ground Rules – Sometimes Known as Establishing a 'Holding Environment'

- Being the focus of attention for some people can be extraordinarily uncomfortable.
- Being clear about the expectations of coaching, setting ground rules, and finding a safe and private space for discussion is essential. In busy working environments, these are going to be even harder to find and yet sacred to protect.
- A coachee is likely to reveal personal experiences, resulting in a potential sense of vulnerability; being aware of this is crucial in developing trust and rapport with students/coachees.
- We all react in different ways and being mindful of the sensitivities to your reaction, as a coach, is crucial. Keeping mindful of an individual's vulnerability is essential to the coaching relationship that you are hoping will grow.

Assumption Three: Unconscious Emotional Reactivity and Recovery

It is crucial for a coach to expand their colleague's capacity for self-regulation emotionally, where feelings can be expressed safely and without fear of judgement.

- Verbalising feelings can help an individual find ways and means to manage themselves more helpfully. When we look at cognitive behaviour coaching, some of these tools enable that process of examining and managing emotions simply and powerfully.
- Emotional intelligence competences. Goleman in his work on leadership (Goleman et al. 2002; Goleman 2006) identified an impressive list of attributes that help manage our emotional reactivity and include:
  1. self-awareness
  2. self-regulation
  3. motivation
  4. empathy
  5. social skills.

Goleman (in Bird and Gornall 2016: p. 52) argues that the greater insight we have into ourselves the more likely we are to be able to manage our emotional responses effectively.

Rogers (2012: p. 260) reflects on the emotional intelligence model but raises the key maturity needed to process our experiences, our emotions, and our learning. What really appeals to me, as a coach, is the opportunity to share this information with my colleagues in order to reflect and discuss the impact these ideas have on our practice as coaches.

The more mindful we are of our responses, the more likely we are to take our time in responding to others. By being more careful in our responses, we may be less impulsive; thereby encouraging a calm and engaging response to difficult situations, rather than flying off the handle with potentially unhelpful results. As those involved with potentially life and death situations in your everyday work, this self-awareness is crucial to creating the calmness needed to care and support each other as well as your patients.

Assumption Four: Defence

Some patterns of behaviour – such as denial, blame, and projection – emerge when we become uncomfortable and defensive, finding the emotions too difficult to handle.

- Issues such as projection, transference, and counter-transference can be explored carefully with some reference to their origins, but if past experiences of trauma have been buried, then referral is always an important consideration and should follow organisational policy. Coaching supervision is a crucial support to the coach in identifying what may be needed when tricky issues arise and referral is needed.
- Drawing on some useful tools to develop self-awareness, such as the drama triangle (Karpman in Bird and Gornall 2016: p. 54) as well as the positive antidote with the use of the winner's triangle (Choy in Bird and Gornall 2016: p. 60).

Cognitive Behavioural Coaching

To put it simply, how we think (based on our memories, experience, and assumptions) determines how we feel and how we behave. There is evidence to suggest that this also impacts on our physiology or health. As health practitioners we need all the help we can get to manage our health and that of those we work with.

The insightful work of cognitive behaviour coaches Palmer, Dryden, and Edgerton (in Palmer and Whybrow 2008) have led to the development of practical tools and training in ways of supporting cognitive behaviour coaching. They encourage self-research and self-monitoring as ways for people to help themselves in order to challenge and build more positive ways of thinking, feeling, and acting. The process can potentially help students move towards becoming the kind of person they want to be, attaining outcomes desired personally and professionally.

This communicates the holistic and in-depth approach that cognitive behaviour coaching can offer both to ourselves and to those we coach. The cognitive approach manages to offer not only practical problem solving but also an opportunity to overcome all sorts of obstacles: emotional, psychological, and behavioural. When students present with issues such as self-harming, loss of confidence, and extreme anxiety, referral to relevant professional services is crucial.

Edgerton and Palmer's SPACE model (in Palmer and Whybrow 2008: pp. 88–89) offers a comprehensive research route into oneself through examining and researching the Situation, Physiology, Actions, Cognitions, and Emotions. I propose a simpler one – TFA:

Thoughts
Feelings
Action.

One of the reasons I like this approach is the self-sufficiency it offers to the user. Use of this model holds the potential for helping a student improve their own problem solving skills, increasing self-awareness through researching their thoughts and feelings together with the action they choose to take. Ultimately, the coachee undertakes self-coaching.

Let's have a look at what is involved.

As with any coaching, a student will come with an outcome in mind (to manage their workload more effectively/balance the needs of their family life with being a student/ falling out with colleagues/meeting deadlines/being fearful of talking to some patients or undertaking personal care). It may take a while for the rapport to develop between supervisor and student before the student is enabled to vocalise what their goal is. Thoughts are emotionally charged, often linked to past experiences – good and bad –and many people don't realise this about themselves.

Step one: Write the problem out in order to research what is unhelpful (red) and then decide what might be more helpful (green) using the following headings:

Thoughts

It's distressing for my patients to be undressed by a stranger

I will hurt them by mistake

I am always gentle and careful when I touch patients

Feelings

I feel embarrassed and anxious

Fear of hurting them

Proud of my approach

Actions

I avoid doing intimate patient care and leave it to my colleagues where possible

Defensive and grumpy with colleagues

Be as gentle and respectful as I can with patients I care for

Volunteer to support colleagues when I see them struggling

The supervisor offers some challenge when the red data is collected:

- What are you assuming?
- What is the evidence you are basing this on?
- When has this happened?

The coachee can see that a feeling is different from a thought and the evidence behind the thought can be explored.

Working on this together is a form of collaboration. You as the supervisor are genuinely curious, helping the student to surface some unhelpful thoughts, feelings, and actions. This sort of collaboration has the potential of bringing the supervisor and student closer together in a shared viewing, writing, and talking activity, so it engages a lot of senses; touch, sound, sight, and feeling. For students who have dyslexia, this may be an excellent opportunity to use all the student's senses – visual, verbal reasoning, self-reflection – it may also offer an opportunity for the student to carry out some self-reflection and processing in their own time.

A student commits to the act of writing their thoughts down – perhaps for the first time. The difference between what is said and what is written down is a great map. You see what the student is shying away from. It's usually quite important.

This kinaesthetic representation of articulating what is going on inside an individual's head can be particularly attractive to the visual learner. Experimenting with using coloured pens to depict the processes involved – e.g. blue for initial prospecting, red for hot or unhelpful, and green for more helpful – can engage learners in a way that recognises their preferred learning style.

This introduction to TFA may be the first time a student has thought about how their thoughts and feelings link to affect their actions. They may also start to surface any core beliefs or assumptions they are making. This in turn provides self-awareness and insight on the impact of any thinking errors.

Thinking errors to be aware of as a coach, educator, or student

Thinking errors are where an individual focuses on insufficient or unreliable data drawing illogical conclusions without any substantive evidence (based on the work of Curwen et al. 2007: p. 130). Identifying thinking errors can be a powerful means to securing greater self-management in terms of the coachees' well-being. We all commonly use thinking errors and they include the following:

All or nothing thinking: They are all against me!

Magnification/awfulising: There is nothing that can ever happen to help me now!

Minimisation: It was nothing!

Personalisation: It's always my fault!

Emotional reasoning: I know this will be a disaster!

Mind reading/jumping to conclusions: I know exactly what he is thinking!

Labelling: It's the number-crunching sceptics from management again who do not understand our core business!

Discounting the positives: I realised she was just saying that to get to her next meeting – she didn't mean it!

Mental filter/focus on the negative: As soon as he sees me he remembers what happened last time!

Demands: I would have thought she should have remembered what I said to him yesterday about how I was feeling!

Fortune telling/catastrophising: I know what's going to happen now and it's all going to be a disaster!

Low frustration tolerance levels: I can't stand this anymore I'm leaving!

Phoneyism: My tutor can see through my lack of knowledge and they don't trust me!

Blame: I really shouldn't have been expected to do this job!

Having an awareness that these thinking errors exist in us all helps us to self-monitor and manage them out of our heads, either in a self-coaching style or in a coaching conversation.

It is difficult to challenge assumptions or core beliefs, so great sensitivity is needed. Questions such as 'what will that mean to you?' and then 'what does that say about you?' may help you to discover these core beliefs. The troublesome thought is often as a result of a troublesome core belief or assumption. So, the question 'what if that were true?' can offer the coachee some meaningful acknowledgement and an opportunity to move forward.

Solutions Focused Coaching

This is a favourite approach of mine! Writing this chapter has helped me see how I like to use tools from all the coaching approaches – although like most practitioners I am mainly unaware of what approach I will use until I'm actually with the person. I will listen carefully and, depending on what they say or feel about a situation that they find themselves in, only then will this data direct me to the tool I use.

The solutions focused approach is very much about encouraging the person to describe their problem resolved – in other words how they would like things to be – their desired outcome achieved. This conversation enables them to get into a more positive place and in doing so they begin to see what is needed to achieve a solution. Solutions emerge from the coachee/student, not from you the coach/supervisor. As Rogers (2012: p. 280) so clearly communicated:

> It is far more important for the individual to gain insight into themselves than for you to do so.

Rogers goes on to quote from Carl Jung's book *Modern Man in Search of a Soul* (Jung 1933), which given the context of this book, is even more eye catching:

> Nothing is more unbearable for the patient than to always be understood. It is relatively unimportant whether the psychotherapist understands or not, but everything hangs on the patient doing so.

When a woman gives birth, she becomes a patient of sorts, except that normally she is well and needs the support and knowledge of midwives to help in the process of giving birth. This relationship is crucial to not just the success of the birth but also the confidence of the parent going forward with her baby in the future. It is advisable then, as professionals, to invest in understanding ourselves, although invariably this can be challenging!

The OSCAR model (Rogers et al. 2012 : 5) is a great template used in solutions focused coaching and is a great help for productive meetings either in teams, or in one-to-ones:

> Getting people to look forward to what they want to be doing in the future is reflective of the nature of solutions focused coaching. After defining the desired Outcome or Destination we encourage people to look at where they are starting from, the present.

Outcome – Destination	What would make this conversation of greatest value?
	What is the problem?
	What would success look like?
Situation – the starting point	Tell me more about what is going on?
	What is currently happening?
	Who is involved?
	What makes it an issue now?
Choices and consequences – the route options	What have you already tried?
	What choices do you feel you have? Outline what you think are the consequences of each choice?
	Which choices have the best consequences?

Action – the detailed plan	What action will you take?
	How will you take it?
	Who will take it and by when?
	How motivated on a scale of 1–10 do you feel to take the actions?
Review – Making sure you are on track!	What steps will you take to review your progress?
	How far are the actions moving you towards your outcome?
	When will we review the outcomes of the action?

Person-Centred Coaching

Carl Rogers during the 1940s and 1950s promoted the person-centred stance advocating that people were their own experts. This belief was a contradiction to previously held beliefs contained in behaviourism and psychoanalysis, where it was assumed that experts knew what was best for their clients. The non-directive influence of Rogers had begun, and coaching reflects this philosophical approach where person-centred coaching is not **what** you do, but **how** you do it (Joseph and Linley 2006b in Cox et al. 2014: 69)

- The person-centred approach comes from a philosophical approach often linked or associated with an impressive term: 'unconditional positive regard'– where you genuinely and whole-heartedly believe in the person you are working with, to resolve his or her problems.
- Using your skills in reflective listening, the coach or trainer develops empathic understanding of the coachee or student's internal world, in order to help them makes sense of their own situation and resolve issues for themselves, rather than be directed to action.
- There are times when this is the same for the patient: if everything is going well then the patient can exercise greater control over their birth experience, but if either mother or baby are in danger then a more directive approach is needed.

- The coach has to trust their client to find his or her own direction in life and to maintain an empathic, genuine unconditional positive regard throughout their work together. Think about what will help you to maintain this and what support you might need.
- Skills and performance coaching, which is very much the focus of this book, requires the skills and commitment of the coach to achieving high levels of performance in empathy. Let's just distinguish between sympathy and empathy:

  Sympathy is in essence feeling sorry for someone else. It does not imply supporting them to achieve their potential or change in any way, rather it is a process of identifying or sharing someone else's feelings which can in turn lead to projection or transference. Sympathy can result unintentionally in sending a message that you feel sorry for the person you are working with, that they are somehow less equal, and you perceive them as a victim rather than capable and resourceful. Taking on the emotions of others is exhausting and should really be done by counsellors or therapists who are specially trained.

  Empathy on the other hand does not mean that you feel the same as the person you are working with, but that you are trying to understand how they feel and view the world through their eyes, rather than yours. There are times when you need to make a personal connection to build rapport, but you still need to stay resourceful in order to act professionally and be of use to your students.

Gestalt and Coaching

Founded in Germany in the early twentieth century by Fritz and Laura Perls (Perls et al. 1951) this radical holistic view of the human mind translated means 'form'. It is based on the idea that the mind has the capacity to put things together and view them as a whole. So, unlike experimental psychology where everything is dissected in detail, this encourages the coachees to look at themselves as part of a bigger picture.

One of the helpful tools I have found from this approach as a coach is also associated with Neuro Linguistic Programming (NLP), which can be described as the study of the structure of subjective experience and can be considered as still evolving in application alongside other therapies such as hypnosis.

Promoted by Seier (in Cox et al. 2014: p. 109), this offers some excellent questions for us to experiment with.

- What is at stake for you here?
- What is missing that is important for you?
- What is not being taken care of that matters to you?

Narrative Coaching

David Drake (in Wildflower and Brennan 2011: p. 273) is a prolific writer on the narrative approach to coaching. There is quite a complex development of the approach, but the important thing to remember is that we all have our own stories 'drawn from a rich tapestry of historical, contextual, and mythical narratives' (Drake in Wildflower and Brennan 2011: p. 271)

The stories often shift as we attempt to interact and relate well or influence others. Working with other people's stories as a coach helps people to:

1. Become more aware of their unconscious – making explicit the implicit.
2. Recognise the impact the stories have on behaviour and identity.
3. Look at how these stories were built and the assumptions made.
4. Offer the possibility of role invention and creation of a new story!

Psychological Development in Adulthood and Coaching

Essentially what comes under this big heading is theory and research about developmental changes in our psychological make up and how this impacts on our practice of coaching.

Watching out for the potential impact of a mid-life crisis is what this may come down to in terms of coaching. Yearnings for unfulfilled dreams can result in all sorts of complications for an individual and often reading what others have done to overcome this helps to reassure the individual that they are not alone and may help dissolve feelings of frustration, anger, or shame. Being reminded that this is not a permanent state may also help the individual.

Whilst Vailant's (in Palmer and Whybrow 2008) and Erikson's (in Cox et al. 2014) adult development stages are of some interest, like with any model they are just a launch pad for reflective listening, questioning, and potential action.

Wildflower and Brennan (2011:p. 42) list these stages as:

1. *Intimacy* versus *isolation.*
2. *Career consolidation* versus *self-absorption.*
3. *Generativity* versus *stagnation.*
4. *Keeper of the meaning* versus *rigidity.*
5. *Integrity* versus *despair.*

Understanding these stages can help you gain insight into where your coachee/student may be coming from and a relief for your coachee/student in terms of explaining the reason they are experiencing these unhelpful thoughts.

Using Kegan and Lahey's (2001) immunity to change process will potentially help an individual to uncover what they perceive to be 'competing commitments' and 'big assumptions' that hold us all back from making key changes. Our unhelpful assumptions can also be identified and dealt with when using the SPACE or TFA models in cognitive behaviour coaching. Making explicit our thinking errors gives us all a chance to challenge and correct them through coaching.

Positive Psychology

This is the science of well-being and optimal functioning. Looking at positive emotions, building resilience or 'bouncebackability' – as Pemberton (2015) describes it, strengths, and flow. Csikszentmihalyi and Seligman (2000) argue that there are three sources of happiness:

1. Experiencing pleasure.
2. Meaning in life.
3. Experiencing 'flow' at work or play: no worries; being completely involved in what you are doing.

Being resilient … bouncebackability

Carole Pemberton's (2015) work on resilience is extensive but with my coaching hat on I am choosing her 4S model as one to help students, as well the coach or educator, at times of crisis.

Skills & Qualities	Strategies – Action
What are you most proud of in terms of the skills you have?	What are the approaches you take?
How would you describe yourself to someone?	Rearranging things that can be put off if stressful and doing what is most important or most urgent etc. Managing diary.
Feedback?	
Supports	**Sagacity – Wisdom**
What keeps you going when you are having a really tough day?	What are the sayings and learnings that have been handed to you that you remember to help you?
They can be anchors/people etc.	

Transactional Analysis

Transactional analysis (TA) is often used in conversations, as people have been made aware through media and education of this popular humanistic approach that can be argued to offer optimism about human nature and development (Napper and Newton in Cox et al. 2014: p. 170).

- *People are OK.*
- *Everyone can think.*
- *Therefore people can decide to change if they wish.*

Eric Berne in the 1960s and 1970s with his book *The Games People Play* (1964) created awareness of TA, it's assumptions and principles and, as Rogers in Wildflower and Brenan (Wildflower and Brennan 2011:p. 29) outline, these assumptions and principles underpin our coaching approach today. The following table brings together the foundation assumptions of TA and coaching principles as outlined by Jenny Rogers (2012). Whilst there is some room for discussion and disagreement, the over-riding learning is the way in which the assumptions are so closely aligned with the principles of coaching.

Ego states have a complex narrative but can and have been simply expressed as:

Adult – neutral – argued as our rational self where we are non-judgmental and in our most logical of states.

Parent – often replaying behaviours we have learned from key figures in our past. This is where we find our self-discipline and therefore it is characterised by guilt and 'should'. Also often broken down in to nurturing and controlling states with related behaviours.

Child –again a state where we replay observed behaviour, which may encompass creativity and joy – the natural child – playful and spontaneous. Alternatively, there is the adapted or wilful child: sulky, obedient, and reluctantly compliant.

We all have all of these ego states playing out in our everyday lives to a larger or lesser degree and the TA assumptions link with coaching principles.

TA assumption (Rogers in Wildflower and Brennan 2011: pp. 29–30)	Coaching principles (Rogers 2012: pp. 7–9)
People are OK. You are OK and I'm OK – I accept what you do even if I don't agree with it. Equals regardless of difference and status.	Principle 1 Rogers 2012: p. 7
	The client is resourceful.
	Essentially this refers to how the client has all the answers they need inside them and your job as the coach is to help them think more powerfully as to how they can resolve issues or challenges for themselves.
You have a choice – you are the most powerful influencer in your life!	Principle 3 Rogers 2012: p. 8
	Coaching addresses the whole person – past, present ,and future; work and private lives!
	There are often sources of pain and difficulties in any individual's life and whilst some of these cannot be changed we can all change how we respond to them.

Practitioner–client relationships are based on equality. We work as equals.	Principle 5 Rogers 2012: p. 9 The coach and coachee are equals. Total respect is needed for you to work in collaboration as two adults.
There is open and transparent communication where TA is taught and used positively and constructively to assist the coachee to be even more aware of their choices and action needed.	Principle 2 Rogers 2012: p. 8 The coach's role is to develop the client's resourcefulness through skilful questioning, challenge, and support.
Everyone has the capacity to think. You are responsible for yourself and you live with the consequences of your decisions.	Principle 4: the client sets the agenda.

Some Conclusions

The potential for helping learners or coaches is more important than the origin of the model used. Some coaches get stuck in a rut using a model they feel comfortable with, not necessarily a model that could help the person they are working with. With the help of regular self-assessment and reflection, client feedback and review, supported with regular supervision, you can keep working on your skills and energy to be the best for the students you are supporting.

The best way of developing your skill and confidence as a coach is to just to have a go at using reflective listening first; open and probing questions next. The content-free questions set out later in this chapter are an excellent starting point for anyone having a go at coaching.

Reflective practice is a key component of any professional's life and it is a necessity in developing competence and confidence in a coach.

- After each session, take a minute to carry out a brief assessment of how you felt you got on.
- What went well?
- What would you do differently next time?
- What have you learnt as a result?

Our best learning is often when we get things wrong. One of the ways I got started in developing my coaching skills was to turn off the attention on me and focus on listening. I found this really tiring at first – listening reflectively to others requires you to park yourself and focus only on the other person. The more you practise, the more it becomes second nature; you can then practise using those 'content-free open questions'. Always ask for feedback and start to note down your progress. These simple but super powerful skills will soon make the difference you want to make!

Key coaching skills and templates to experiment with:

What is coaching?

'helping others discover their own wisdom'

What coaching is	What coaching isn't
Conversations, techniques, and action plans aimed at helping the person to improve, develop, learn new skills, find personal success, achieve aims, and manage life change and personal challenges.	The coach imposing a template for the person on how to live their life, fix their problems, etc.
Non-judgemental.	The coach sitting in judgement on the person.
Careful attentive listening to their wants and concerns.	The coach talking at the person.
A process that identifies and uses the person's own resources to help them move forward.	The coach telling the person what to do.
The coach helping the person to do their own thinking and generate their own options for action.	The coach giving direction and steering the person.
Helping the person find their own solutions	The coach doing things for the person.

A solutions focused approach to coaching includes the GROW model as promoted by John Whitmore (2009).

Goal	What specifically do you want to achieve?
Reality	What is happening now?
Options	What else could you try?
Will do	What is the first thing you will do?

The OSCAR model was formulated by British coaches and trainers Andrew Gilbert and Karen Whittleworth (Rogers et al., 2012).

OUTCOME The destination	What would make today's session of greatest value?
SITUATION The starting point	What is currently happening?
CHOICES AND CONSEQUENCES The route options	What are your choices and which have the best consequences?
ACTIONS The detailed plan	What will you do and when will you do it?
REVIEW Making sure you are on track	What steps will you take to review your progress?

Content-free questions. Based on Rogers (2012: p. 85)

1. What's the issue?
2. What makes it an issue now?
3. Who owns this issue?
4. How important, on a scale of 1–10, is this?
5. How much, on a scale of 1–10, do you want to solve this?
6. Tell me about the implications of doing nothing?
7. What have you already tried?
8. Visualise the problem solved. Tell me what would be happening that is not happening now?
9. What is preventing the ideal outcome?
10. What is your responsibility for what has been happening?
11. What are the early signs of things getting better?
12. At your most resourceful, what might you say to yourself or someone else?
13. What are you options for action?
14. What criteria will you use to judge these actions?
15. Which option is the best?
16. What is the first step?

17. When will you take it?
18. What does that mean to you?
19. What will be helpful?
20. Avoid 'Why …' and 'but…'.

References

Berne, E. (1964). *Games People Play: The Psychology of Human Relationships*. London: Penguin.

Bird, J. and Gornall, S. (2016). *The Art of Coaching: A handbook of tips and tools Abingdon*. Routledge.

Cox, E., Bachkirova, T., and Clutterbuck, D. (2014). *The complete Handbook of Coaching*, 2e. Ashford: Sage.

Csikszentmihalyi, M. and Seligman, M.E. (2000). Positive psychology: an introduction. *American Psychologist* 55 (1): 5–14.

Curwen, B., Palmer, S., and Ruddell, P. (2007). *Brief Cognitive Behaviour Therapy. Ashford*. Sage.

Freud, S. (1922). *Introductory Lectures on Psychoanalysis*. London: Routledge.

Goleman, D. (2006). The socially intelligent. *Educational Leadership* 64 (1): 76–81.

Goleman, D., Boyatzis, R., and McKee (2002). *Primal leadership: Realizing the power of emotional intelligence*. Harvard Business School Press.

Jung, C.G. (1933). *Modern Man in Search of a Soul*, trans. *WS Dell and Cary F*. In: *Baynes*. New York and London: Harcourt Brace Jovanovich.

Jung, C.G. (1956). *Symbols of Transformation: The Collected Works of CG Jung*. Routledge & Kegan Paul.

Kegan, R. and Lahey, L. (2001). *How We Talk Can Change the Way We Work: Seven Languages for Transformation*. San Franscisco: Jossey-Bass.

Kline, N. (2015). *More Time to Think*. London: Cassel.

Kolb, D. (1984). *Experiential Learning: Experience as the Source of Learning and Development*. Upper Saddle River, NJ: Prentice Hall.

Palmer and Whybrow (2008). *Handbook of Coaching Psychology*. London and New York: Routledge.

Pemberton, C. (2015). *Resilience: A Practical Guide for Coaches*. McGraw-Hill.

Perls, F., Hefferline, G., and Goodman, P. (1951). *Gestalt Therapy: Excitement and Growth in the Human Personality*. Julian Press.

Rogers, J. (2012). *Coaching Skills - a handbook*, 3e. Maidenhead: Open University Press.

Rogers, J., Whittleworth, K., and Gilbert, A. (2012). *Manager as Coach*. Maidenhead: McGraw-Hill.

Siegel, D.J. (2010). *Mindsight: The New Science of Personal Transformation*. Bantam.

Whitmore, J. (2009). *Coaching for Performance: 4th edition: GROWing human potential and purpose*. London: Brealey.

Wildflower, L. and Brennan, D. (2011). *The Handbook of Knowledge-Based Coaching: From Theory to Practice*. San Francisco: Jossey-Bass.

6

Evaluation

There have been a number of evaluations of the CLiP™ model in the UK and in writing this book we wanted to provide an opportunity for the study authors to provide some detail of their work without replicating the published papers. Studies were supported by funding from Health Education England (HEE) for University of East Anglia (UEA) and Plymouth University. In this chapter, the authors provide their commentary on their own studies.

Collaborative Learning in Practice: Coaching to Support Student Learners in Healthcare, First Edition. Charlene Lobo, Rachel Paul, and Kenda Crozier.
© 2021 John Wiley & Sons Ltd. Published 2021 by John Wiley & Sons Ltd.
Companion website: www.wiley.com/go/lobo/collaborativelearninginpractice

6.1

Plymouth University

Graham Williamson, Adele Kane and Jane Bunce

Background

The School of Nursing and Midwifery at Plymouth University engages with placement providers across Somerset, Devon, and Cornwall. As part of our regional project to implement Collaborative Learning in Practice (CLiP™) in hospital and community settings, we undertook a programme of research activity, most of which was funded by HEE. This chapter reports on three of the research studies in detail and a fourth in brief. These studies were: a systematic review of the literature, two qualitative studies (one in hospital and another in community nursing settings), with a fourth examining whether or not increasing student nurse numbers in placements in CLiP makes a difference to patient safety.

It is important for nurse education placement learning that policy change has an appropriate evidence base to provide the foundation for today's nursing courses and placement learning experiences to meet the expectations of the NMC's Future Nurse Standards (NMC 2018a). Without an evidence base, initiatives run the risk of piecemeal implementation, with certain features being adopted and others omitted – and different specifications and terminology in different areas. The original conception of CLiP with related nomenclature is being implemented in the UK, and whilst this indicates the willingness of educational institutions and practice partners to innovate, it also makes it difficult to evaluate the success or otherwise of these initiatives. For example, the following terms are all current in the UK, with clinical areas using 'collaborative learning in clusters' (CLIC); 'the Salford Model'; 'coaching and peer assisted learning' (C-PAL; Wareing et al. 2018); 'collaborative assessment and learning' (CALM); 'CLIP-style model'. All of these appear distinct from the 'Amsterdam model', CLiP's origin; and are more removed from coaching approaches, which are also numerous, with distinct overlaps with CLiP. Internationally, Dedicated Education Unit (DDE) may be a similar means of placement learning, but this is speculative given the diversity of application of terminology that we found in the literature (Williamson et al. 2020c). In view of these features and an emerging literature on this subject, our first study – a systematic review of the literature – was important to scope existing research.

Study 1: Collaborative Learning in Practice: A Systematic Review and Narrative Synthesis of the Research Evidence in Nurse Education

We conducted a thorough, rigorous systematic review of the literature on CLiP to discover whether there was a research evidence base for claims relating to peer support, accelerated learning, and improvements in registered practice (Williamson et al. 2020c).

The question this systematic review sought to answer is: 'What is the evidence for effectiveness of CLiP models?' The search strategy was derived using PICO: Population was 'student (undergraduate, baccalaureate) nurses'; Intervention was 'CLiP models'; Comparison was 'other models of placement learning'; Outcome was 'any relevant'. We deliberately sought to include research studies from any methodology. This systematic review protocol was registered with PROSPERO (CRD42018106838).

A comprehensive search was undertaken between October and December 2018 using a variety of search terms that followed on from the PICO. We will not report the process in its entirety here because it is covered in the full paper (Williamson et al. 2020c). Searches were undertaken in CINAHL, MEDLINE, ERIC, NICE, EMBASE, COCHRANE, CRD, JBI, Grey Literature (including manual Search and SINGLE), US clinical trials.gov, ISRCTN registry of clinical trials, Ethos, Google Scholar. This initial work garnered 1335 hits, which were narrowed down by scrutiny for relevance to 204. These were read in detail, which left 18 papers for quality appraisal independently by the research team, who scored the papers, discussed them, and agreed those to be included in the synthesis. This process left 14 papers for inclusion.

The results of the literature search indicate that there is no body of literature relating specifically to the use of CLiP models. Only one study (Hill et al. 2016) discusses systematic evaluation of CLiP, but that was unpublished at that time in a peer reviewed journal – although this has subsequently been rectified (Hill et al. 2020). The 14 papers we found were about the DDE concept, and we conducted a narrative synthesis of them. Key findings support the assertions related to Collaborative Learning in Practice, albeit in different models of placement learning.

Since this review was completed, a number of other teams have published important research in this area. For example, a team from UEA (Hill et al. 2020) have published data from their seminal study from 2015, which was included in our review as a report (Hill et al. 2016). This was previously only available in report form. Their findings are expertly summarised in their paper and, as we will see below, chime with our own analyses. Hill et al. (2020) use a mixed methods design, with data from the Clinical Learning Environment Inventory (CLEI; Shivers et al. 2017), and found students who had experienced CLiP reported lower supervisory relationship scores compared with those without experience, a similar pedagogical atmosphere in placements with two themes emerging form the qualitative data ('Adapting the environment' and 'Learning to fly'). They report CLiP to offer many benefits as an approach to clinical learning but note that attention needs to be paid to ensuring sufficient numbers of students, and potential losses as well as gains. Working with UEA colleagues, Harvey and Uren (2019) implemented CLiP in Somerset, and provide some preliminary evidence from one clinical area, indicating that support for placements and clear leadership were essential for gains to be made in CLiP placements.

In summary, our systematic review and subsequent attempts to identify research have proved mostly fruitless and there is little formal evaluation at the time of writing. Conference attendances have indicated that this model is growing in popularity but areas have not yet begun to publish their findings beyond presentations and posters at conferences.

Study 2: 'Thinking like a Nurse'. Changing the Culture of Nursing Students' Clinical Learning: Implementing Collaborative Learning in Practice

This study reports issues concerning the implementation of Collaborative Learning in Practice models at the University of Plymouth School of Nursing and Midwifery, with in-hospital practice partners across the South West of England (Williamson et al. 2020b). We conducted four focus group interviews with 40 students with experience of Collaborative Learning in Practice placements, and two focus groups with eight clinical practice staff with responsibility for implementing and supporting such models in their areas. Data were transcribed and analysed using the Framework Method (Ritchie et al. 2014). Key themes were 'Real-time Practice of Collaborative Learning Implementation', 'Collaborative Learning as Preparation for Registrant Practice', and 'the Student/Mentor Relationship'.

One issue relating to preparation was the perception of change and the need for that to be actively managed. The capacity of CLiP placements increased from perhaps one or two student nurses, up to in some cases 12. Many School of Nursing staff conducted preparation and support activities, including visits to areas where CLiP was already up and running successfully, local workshops, accessing online materials, and teaching sessions for placement staff and students. CLiP was much more successful when clinical staff engaged with this and were prepared to actively manage it:

> The wards put themselves forwards to be chosen for CLiP so there was the buy-in from the start. We had one clinical area who bought into having a Practice Educator to support as a secondment, one day a week. Staff were quite engaged about it. (A staff member)

However, despite introductory sessions provided for students in university and placement locations, these processes appeared not to be remembered, as students described staff and themselves as not aware of the meaning or practice of CLiP:

> I had no idea what CLIP was about at all, so going into it, I didn't know what was to be expected of me and likewise, the staff

members didn't know what was expected of them so, I think there was lack of communication about what the whole procedure was and what was expected of everyone.

It was curious that this response was so widespread amongst students and some staff given the extent and nature of the preparation activities that took place, almost a 'collective amnesia', which has been noted to be prevalent amongst nurses (Moreland et al. 2015). However, it does indicate that change is difficult, close facilitation is necessary at ward/department level, and no doubt when areas have run CLiP more than once, members of staff will understand it better.

Another area of notable success concerned team working. Students articulated greater problem-solving skills by working together and learning from other students, forming lasting friendships:

Seeing the process for us it really does [work] … me and a third year … it gives us a chance to problem solve [for ourselves]. (A second-year student)

Staff made similar remarks about students' collaboration:

I think it worked really well … supporting each other … it's lovely to have them 'cos they really look out for each other. If one [has] a problem, the others are all there sorting it out for them and … they're all interested in each other. (A staff member)

Some students and staff explored the differences between mentoring and coaching, saying:

In the old mentoring style, you're the mentor and the student's behind you, you're protecting them from the work that needs doing but now with CLIP, you're putting the student in front of you and expecting them to do their job, and it's come as a shock to some of them … A second-year student said to me [at the beginning of a CLIP placement] 'They've given me a patient to look after'; I said 'yeah, that sounds like a really good idea'. (A staff member)

Whilst a student noted:

[My mentor] said 'I've got to learn to stand back and let you just get on with it' … it's a new thing for them as well, sometimes they forget and so have to remind themselves to stand back. It's hard 'cos they're used to just getting on with it themselves. (A student)

Our findings in this first empirical study indicate that the key issues were how CLiP facilitated students' learning through 'real-time' practice, helped them to prepare for registrant practice, and altered the student–mentor relationship to one more akin to coaching and the assessor–supervisor relationship in the revised NMC (2018b) standards. Our 'real-time' theme resonates with the work of others (Hill et al. 2020), and will contribute to greater 'work readiness' at point of registration (Wolff et al. 2010).

Study 3: Investigating the Implementation of a Collaborative Learning in a Practice Model of Nurse Education in a Community Placement Cluster: A Qualitative Study

Attracting new graduate nurses to work in the community is problematic, and this has contributed to shortages in this sector in the United Kingdom and internationally (Williamson et al. 2020a). With this in mind, we trialled CLiP in a pilot study in our region, with the intention to increase placement capacity, introduce students to this sector, and accelerate their learning and development of key skills and behaviours. We were specifically interested in the views of student nurses and the staff, supporting them on placement about their experiences of implementing CLiP, because community settings are so different from in-hospital settings and we were keen to learn lessons that might have an impact on future development of placements and placement capacity in the community. In this study, students were placed in three settings: three nursing homes (although one withdrew), two hospices, and two general practitioner (GP) health centres with GP nurses.

We conducted four focus group interviews between winter 2018 and spring 2019, with 31 staff and students in two English counties in the South West of England. These were transcribed and analysed using the

Framework Method; themes were discussed and agreed by the research team. What we found was quite interesting, and was both similar and different to the previous study (Williamson et al. 2020b), which was conducted in-hospital. Three themes emerged: 'Peer support', which concerned the benefits of being in placement with other students; 'Developing and learning', which was about the acquisition of skills including leadership; and 'Organisation', which related to issues and concerns involved in the preparation and daily management of the CLiP experience. There were some positive quotes about peer support, for example:

> Peer learning has been quite beneficial because the second years taught the third years some stuff as well and you know, just because everyone has different placements so I think that's been really beneficial just learning from each other and different experiences and you know, different ways to change dressings and things. (A student)

> I've learnt from the third years. I've learnt an awful lot from the third years not as 'this is how you do this' and not communication skills, but management and you just learn from each other don't you. (Another student)

However, there were some negative comments from the nursing home setting about conflicts with students, and these came from staff as well as students.

> We kept getting told that they'd had students previously and they stopped having them for a while because they were 'too posh to wash' and so … we felt we had to prove ourselves as HCAs (which is not what we're there for) and we were worried [to progress towards registration]. (A student)

Staff also noted potential conflict in one setting:

> There were a couple of instances where the students, the power of numbers, they become quite intimidating amongst themselves – they were quite forceful, it made them quite forceful characters … we've had a couple of instances where we've

had to address that and challenge that and I don't think that would've happened in a traditional –mentorstudent model. (A staff member)

Overall, this study was successful in addressing its primary aim, which was to investigate issues related to the implementation of CLiP in the community sector, specifically nursing homes, hospices, and GP practice settings. This is an important study internationally because it relates to the exposure of student nurses to community nursing, including increases in placement capacity, which may go some way to ameliorate nursing shortages in that sector. We note that staff and students' perceptions of CLiP concepts differed according to the area in which they were working. Students and staff working in the nursing home sector were generally more negative in their perceptions, with students struggling to connect their nursing care activities with potential registrant practice, and staff reporting conflicts and difficulties. Students in the GP and hospice placements had more of a focus on the clinical skills they developed, the opportunities for complex care (with sick patients in the hospices, and including social prescribing in the GP practices), and activities such as seeing patients in clinics independently (in GP practice, with supervision available but at a distance) and venepuncture. The GP setting's supervision most clearly resembled a coaching model in this respect. Students in this study clearly identified positive views on the extent to which CLiP offered peer support, friendship, and opportunities for peer learning.

Study 4: Student Nurses, Increasing Placement Capacity and Patient Safety. A Retrospective Cohort Study

This study is currently under review with a journal. We were concerned with identifying whether having additional students on placement made any difference to patient safety as defined by metrics from NICE (2014) guidance on safe staffing on falls, pressure ulcers, and medication errors. Logically, it may seem that having more students in placement ought to help with patient safety issues, but concern had been raised in our focus groups (Williamson et al. 2020b) that more students equated to less effective supervision with the potential for errors in care, and some placement staff were unhappy about that potential.

To investigate this issue, using routinely collected audit data on falls, medications errors, and pressure ulcers – anonymised at source from four trusts in our region, we computed risk ratios, mean differences, and correlations to compare outcomes between when placements were running CLiP with three or more students. We received data on 5532 adverse events from 15 clinical areas in four NHS trusts, with 996 students on placement between January 2018 and August 2019. The risk ratio for adverse patient events was favourable when CLiP was operating (RR = 0.9842; 95%; CI 0.9604–1.008), meaning that overall there were 73 less adverse patient events when CLiP was running compared to when it was not. There was a favourable and statistically significant difference in mean adverse patient events ($p = 0.01$; mean difference 279; 95%; CI 213–346) when CLiP was running compared to when it was not. There was no statistically significant correlation between increased student numbers and increased adverse patient events, meaning that having additional students under CLiP did not make patient safety worse on these indicators. Based on this analysis, we conclude that having increased numbers of student nurses in placement during CLiP enhanced patient safety and did not worsen it.

Summary and Key Messages

We conclude that CLiP, utilising models of coaching and peer support, offers benefits to students who are exposed to the reality of nursing practice from the beginning of their placement experiences, enabling them to take greater responsibility and experience heightened peer support than under other previous 'mentoring' arrangements. There are likely to be benefits for nurses supervising and assessing students because these burdens are spread more widely than under one-to-one mentorship models. The potential for developing supportive friendships with other students is important and should not be underestimated as a factor helping students to stay in programmes of study (Williamson et al. 2013): it is axiomatic that where a placement area has several students learning together, this potential is increased. This was a similar message in hospital and community settings. We had not anticipated the less positive finding concerning the potential for 'horizontal violence' about which we speculated in relation particularly to nursing home placements (Williamson et al. 2020a). CLiP is the subject of multiple assertions concerning potential benefits. Our qualitative research supports some of these assertions in some areas, but more work needs to be done to quantify them. We have shown that patient safety is enhanced with additional students; we need to establish if there are any links between CLiP and patient care improvements – research which we are currently planning. Other researchers are also beginning to publish about their CLiP experiences, illustrating benefits for students including leadership skills development, exposure to the real world of nursing, and a greater sense of autonomy for decision making (Harvey and Uren 2019; Hill et al. 2020). We are hopeful, therefore, that this method of placement learning will develop a strong evidence base to inform and support future implementation.

References

Harvey, S. and Uren, C.D. (2019). Collaborative learning: application of the mentorship model for adult nursing students in the acute placement setting. *Nurse Education Today* 74: 38–40.

Hill, R., Woodward, M. and Arthur, A. (2016). Collaborative Learning in Practice (CLiP): Evaluation Report. University of Easy Anglia and Health Education East of England.

Hill, R., Woodward, M., and Arthur, A. (2020). Collaborative learning in practice (CLIP): evaluation of a new approach to clinical learning. *Nurse Education Today* 85: 104295.

Moreland, J.J., Ewoldsen, D.R., Albert, N.M. et al. (2015). Predicting nurses' turnover: the aversive effects of decreased identity, poor interpersonal communication, and learned helplessness. *Journal of Health Communication* 20 (10): 1155–1165.

National Institute for Health and Care Excellence (2014). Safe staffing for nursing in adult inpatient wards in acute hospitals. Safe staffing guideline [SG1] NICE. London: National Institute for Health and Care Excellence.

Nursing and Midwifery Council (2018a). *Future Nurse: Standards of Proficiency for Registered Nurses*. London: Nursing and Midwifery Council.

Nursing and Midwifery Council (2018b). Realising professionalism. Standards for education and training. Part 2: Standards for student supervision and assessment. London: Nursing and Midwifery Council.

Ritchie, J., Lewis, J., Nicholls, C.M., and Ormston, R. (2014). *Qualitative Research Practice: A Guide for Social Science Students and Researchers*, 2e. London: SAGE.

Shivers, E., Hasson, F., and Slater, P. (2017). Pre-registration nursing student's quality of practice learning: clinical learning environment inventory (actual) questionnaire. *Nurse Education Today* 55: 58–64.

Wareing, M., Green, H., Burden, B. et al. (2018). "Coaching and peer-assisted learning" (C-PAL) - the mental health nursing student experience: a qualitative evaluation. *Journal of Psychiatric and Mental Health Nursing* 25 (8): 486–495.

Williamson, G.R., Health, V., and Proctor-Childs, T. (2013). Vocation, friendship and resilience: a study exploring nursing student and staff views on retention and attrition. *The Open Nursing Journal* 7 (1): 149.

Williamson, G.R., Bunce, J., Kane, A. et al. (2020a). Investigating the implementation of a collaborative learning in practice model of nurse education in a community placement cluster: a qualitative study. *The Open Nursing Journal* 14 (1): 39–48.

Williamson, G.R., Kane, A., Plowright, H. et al. (2020b). Thinking like a nurse'. Changing the culture of nursing students' clinical learning: implementing collaborative learning in practice. *Nurse Education in Practice* 43: 102742.

Williamson, G.R., Plowright, H., Kane, A. et al. (2020c). Collaborative learning in practice: a systematic review and narrative synthesis of the research evidence in nurse education. *Nurse Education in Practice* 43: 102706.

Wolff, A.C., Pesut, B., and Regan, S. (2010). New graduate nurse practice readiness: perspectives on the context shaping our understanding and expectations. *Nurse Education Today* 30 (2): 187–191.

6.2

University of East Anglia

Antony Arthur, Rebekah Hill and Michael Woodward

Is it Better Than What We Did Before? The Challenge of Evaluating New Models of Practice Learning

There have been many calls for more research and a stronger evidence base for educational interventions in healthcare (Kalb et al. 2015). Yet there is often a sense that new ideas are rapidly rolled out on a wave of enthusiasm, leaving a trail of small retrospective studies in their wake, before the next initiative looms into view on the horizon.

CLiP is a model of practice learning that has been the focus of more research attention than most. The work described by Williamson and colleagues in this chapter reflects that. Educational interventions are notoriously difficult to evaluate. The process of cause and effect is particularly complex in relation to learning. Kirkpatrick's model of educational evaluation (Kirkpatrick and Kirkpatrick 2006) describes four levels of outcomes: reaction (how favourable the training/education was); learning (the depth of learning achieved); behaviour (whether behaviour has changed following intervention); and results (the really tricky bit, which in healthcare means patient outcomes). As the ripple effect extends further from the centre, so it becomes harder to capture the effect or ascribe observed effects to the educational intervention.

The gold standard for any intervention, educational or otherwise, is the randomised controlled trial but this requires (a lot of) money, time, and expertise. It also requires a willingness to accept the end result. There may be no evidence of effectiveness of the new intervention or model, or it may be found to be worse than whatever preceded it. While a trial may not be feasible here, one of the things a trial does is require a well-described intervention – what it is, what it is not, and how it is distinct from what has preceded it. Establishing this is an extremely useful exercise.

In our own study we did not have the time or resource to undertake a trial, but we felt it important to compare those with experience of CLiP to those without. Full details of the study can be found elsewhere (Hill et al. 2020). Interestingly, a number of students were unsure whether or not they had experienced CLiP, a finding also noted by Williamson et al. (Williamson et al. 2020b). This perhaps suggests that at times what feels like a radically different model for educators is not perceived in the same way 'on the ground'. Both qualitative and quantitative data suggested there were losses as well as gains in the movement between a model of mentorship to CLiP. Our use of mixed methods was important – some raw statistics will often tell you something that you cannot look away from. Equally, hearing an authentic voice will bring a highly informative experience to life.

Our experience of evaluating CLiP has taught us a number of things about evaluating complex educational initiatives:

- Think about an evaluation process from the outset.
- Be able to articulate the intervention and be sure that there is a shared understanding across all stakeholders.
- Be prepared to listen to the findings.

The ultimate power of research is not to 'prove things work' but to make things better.

References

Kalb, K.A., O'conner-Von, S.K., Brockway, C. et al. (2015). Evidence-based teaching practice in nursing education: faculty perspectives and practices. *Nursing Education Perspectives* 36: 212–219. https://doi.org/10.5480/14-1472.

Kirkpatrick, D.L. and Kirkpatrick, J.D. (2006). *Evaluating Training Programs*. San Francisco: Berrett-Koehler.

Part II

Coaching Application

7

Introduction to Coaching in Practice

Rachel Paul and Charlene Lobo

In Part 2, we will be examining coaching in practice through the use of case studies and scenarios. Throughout Part 2 we aim to facilitate learning for:

- Supervisors: to create even more productive learning environments that consider both the needs of learners as well as meeting the requirements of the curriculum.
- Students: to increase their awareness of the needs of supervisors and methods of working that use coaching skills to help develop even greater resourcefulness to find solutions and answers for themselves.

The following format will be the basis of Part 2:

Things to think about – here is an opportunity for you to think about and make notes on how you might deal with the situation. This could be an actual experience or a hypothetical proposal on how you might manage such a situation.

Applying theory to practice – discussion on how a coaching approach might apply in this scenario.

Collaborative Learning in Practice: Coaching to Support Student Learners in Healthcare, First Edition. Charlene Lobo, Rachel Paul, and Kenda Crozier.
© 2021 John Wiley & Sons Ltd. Published 2021 by John Wiley & Sons Ltd.
Companion website: www.wiley.com/go/lobo/collaborativelearninginpractice

Exemplar of a coaching conversation – here is an example of a possible conversation pertaining to a specific situation with signposting of the frameworks and theory that underpin the coaching conversation.

 Self-learning – this offers an opportunity for you to reflect on your current practice position:

- As a coach: ask yourself what you need to do as a supervisor to ensure that you can facilitate learning for all your students whilst keeping patient safety foremost.
- As a student: reflect on your learning and note any questions or areas of clarification needed with your supervisor and consider what you could do to become a more effective learner.

 Companion website – we offer further examples and discussion for you to consider on the companion website.

The format of Part 2 is designed so that you keep the notes, reflections, and any learning exercises you undertake to use as evidence of professional development.

Chapter 5 introduced some of the coaching principles and theories we have used in our approaches to coaching in CLiP. In this section we look in detail at some of the key themes we need to consider when we engage in a 'coaching conversation'.

Language of Coaching

The language of coaching underpins all our coaching practice. The coaching conversations we have all very subtly convey our values, beliefs, and judgements of the person and situation by the words we choose, the phrasing, and the tone of our voice. Therefore, as coaches we must always be careful and thoughtful about what we say and how we say it. Coaching focuses on the importance of using a language that helps to create positivity, enhancing motivation and a certain sort of 'can do' attitude; this has the potential to make a real difference to facilitation.

Often when supervising students there can be an automatic tendency to use the *why* question with resulting defensiveness in response.

Supervisor: *Why did you do that?*

What the supervisor really wants to know is the reasoning that the student was using to result in the action taken or to understand the theoretical basis of the reasoning. 'Why' can often appear accusatory or parental. *'Why did you do that when you know you have to do this?'* So, it is best to avoid using the 'why' question when establishing and maintaining an adult-to-adult relationship, where you are building trust and rapport. The other likely result of using 'why' is resulting negativity and tendency for whining! The coaching exemplars give specific examples of how to conduct coaching conversations illustrating the sorts of questioning that provide students with the opportunity to learn and look out for coaching in order to use it for themselves when the situation arises.

The aim of a positive language approach is to move away from defensive responses to a potential 'will do' approach. To suggest there is always change happening and, as health professionals, we can influence that change in our practice by the way we work together – which is an exciting and potentially empowering prospect. There are several ways this can be facilitated:

- Solutions focused conversations (see Chapter 5).
  These focus on an individual's skills, strengths, and qualities that they can use to achieve the outcome they determine or see as needed. The initial meeting between coach and student provides an excellent opportunity for the coach to pick up information on that individual. How best to work with them, what metaphors may work with them, their strengths, qualities, and the values that they reveal. The initial meeting is sometimes called a 'chemistry' meeting or problem free chat where you get to know the individual first. The 'chemistry' may or may not be a luxury that can be afforded. We also believe that it is up to the coach to park his or her feelings as far as possible, as the relationship in coaching needs to be egalitarian. This might pose a challenge in a hierarchical culture. Parking our emotions as a supervisor or coach is crucial to support the practice of reflective listening and the use of clean language where we avoid trying to influence or lead the student.

- Cognitive behaviour coaching conversations (Thoughts, Feelings, Action [TFA]).

As a coach I find undertaking the cognitive behaviour approach is integrated into most coaching conversations I have. As discussed (see Chapter 5), we may have a natural inclination to think the worst of ourselves, usually thinking negative thoughts. If we think something negative based on some faulty thinking this will give rise to unhelpful feelings and actions. Once we have surfaced these as a supervisor and as a student, we have the potential to manage ourselves more positively and productively.

Normally, in a coaching conversation we might use a number of different frameworks for coaching, such as OSCAR (Rogers et al. 2012, pp. 148–149), GROW (Whitmore 2009, p. 56), or perceptual positioning (Palmer and Whybrow 2008, p. 201) to structure our conversations and focus on the student's agenda. However, to explore a point further or get a deeper understanding of the student's perspective, we might integrate a cognitive behaviour approach.

The information we collect from our learners is key to surfacing deeper meanings whilst at the same time communicating empathy and looking for the solution alongside the student. Establishing good rapport and a positive relationship with a student creates an excellent opportunity to build a safe environment where we can probe for the deep meaning behind the statement 'I feel a bit out of my depth', to the specific issue of giving injections, for example. The empathy expressed, having established a good relationship, gives the opportunity to safely challenge unhelpful thoughts, to stimulate more balanced thinking that leads to change and action.

 Below is an exemplar of a coaching conversation using the GROW model as a framework of the conversation and using TFA to explore an issue in more detail.

Thinking, Feeling, and Action conversations in less than 10 minutes:

Signposting theory	Coaching dialogue
Building **rapport** using open questions with genuine interest.	**Coach:** *Good to meet up with you in this first week! How are you finding things so far?*
Evidence of **reflection** on what they are feeling and experiencing suggests an openness.	**Student:** *Well it's a bit of a shock to my system getting here so early and finding my way here on the bus but I think I'm developing a good routine and although I am absolutely exhausted at the end of the day my friends on the course have set up a WhatsApp group and we support each other with little jokes and pictures …*
Sounds helpful is a way of communicating your **active listening.** The student is realising benefits from initial colleagues' support.	**Coach:** *That sounds helpful to have that background support from others experiencing something similar?*
Genuine positive curiosity, exploring thoughts communicated in open questioning – adult-to adult-openness in communication.	**Student:** *Absolutely! It's got me out of a pickle on a couple of occasions where I couldn't remember where I was supposed to be or what I was meant to be doing!*
Student clearly feels they can trust the supervisor to reveal very quickly the concerns they have.	**Coach:** *Great! So, tell me more about what has been going well with the community placement?*
Focusing on the feelings is crucial in building trust and openness	**Student:** *I feel a bit out of my depth there.*
	Coach: *Tell me more about what it is making you feel out of your depth?*
The student is clearly discounting anything positive and focusing only on the negatives – **thinking error**	**Student:** *Well everything.*
	Coach: *Everything?*
Time for a **challenge**	**Student:** *ok well not everything. I really like the patients I have met and they seem really friendly to me. It's just that I don't seem to be confident with injections.*
The student is starting to manage his/her thoughts more positively and indicates that he/she enjoys being with the patients and the problem is giving injections	**Coach:** *That sounds like you have built really good relationships with your patients what can you do to feel more confident with injections?*
Reflective summary encompassing feelings recognizes the issue	**Student:** *Do more of them? But I don't always know when they are due for the different patients.*
Student encouraged to find solutions and identify action to help him/her help themselves. Student establishes **Goal**: Do more injections. Requests direct observation to check his **reality**	**Coach:** *Doing more is absolutely a good idea! What options do we have to access this?*
Coach encourages student to consider his **options.**	**Student:** *Could I go with other nurses?*
Will do: Student takes ownership of options and action identified with time and place	**Coach:** *I'm sure they would love to take you with them. Let the team know you would like to practice giving injections. How does that feel?*
	Student: *Good – looking forward to getting this sorted!*

Thinking Errors

Thinking errors are something we all suffer from. Essentially, they are the unhelpful thoughts and assumptions we make that may have no evidence to support them but potentially exhaust us by reoccurring in our heads and preventing us from moving forwards. Having awareness that thinking errors exist in us all helps us to self-monitor and manage them out of our heads – either in a self-coaching style or in a coaching conversation. Figure 7.1 is a list of thinking errors we all commonly use based on Palmer and Szymanska (in Palmer and Whybrow 2008: 99)

'Clean' Language

'Clean' language comes from the work of Grove, and his work on using metaphor to express pain as part of the healing process of trauma is well described in Sullivan and Rees (2008). Using the student's metaphors, their language, without any interference in terms of value judgements or assumptions from the coach, you work with the student's values, patterns, issues, and their language. In essence it is avoiding using language that is somehow filled with your agenda or values. Keeping a conversation focused on the student, their needs, and building rapport requires you as the supervisor to take yourself out of the picture and only focus on the student.

Using open questions is key to maintaining focus on the student, it helps the student uncover for themselves their own solution to a particular issue or opportunity they face. The result is potentially greater 'agency' from students, taking self-directed meaning from their learned experiences. Using the principle that the learner sets the agenda, they are driven more by their interests and their agendas rather than just the supervisor's. This may in turn result in increased levels of student ownership for outcomes to be achieved. Self-direction potentially increases confidence to help encourage deeper reflection and engagement with learning. As a result of increased agency, the student may feel more able to overcome potential barriers along the way in their learning journey.

Metaphor is the use of imagery to represent thoughts and feelings. In the above example the student uses the term 'out of my depth' to communicate their depth of emotion and the coach reflects back the same language confirming that they are listening carefully to what is being communicated.

Thinking error	Description	Example	Try this?
All or nothing thinking	Evaluating experiences in extremes/black and white terms/ good or bad.	She is always late. No one ever listens to me.	Challenge 'always' or 'never'. Question what else might be going on here?
Magnification or awfulising: exaggeration	Blowing things out of proportion.	That shift was the worst I have ever done!	Find some middle ground?
Minimisation	Minimising or down playing the part played in a situation.	Anyone could have got a high mark in that exam it was so easy!	What impact is that thinking having on you?
Personalisation	Taking everything personally.	I am responsible for everything and everybody! If that patient dies, it's all my fault!	Write a list of all the other aspects involved with this patient. Who the other people are, the patient's context or circumstances, clarify if you are 100% responsible?
Emotional reasoning	Mistaking thoughts and feelings for facts and not the hypotheses they may be.	I feel like a failure therefore I am one, I feel so nervous I know this procedure will go wrong!	Think more coolly? What would be a more helpful thought? For example: I will do my best! I totally believe this procedure will help this patient to be more comfortable.
Mind reading/ jumping to conclusions	Jumping to a conclusion without the facts or relevant information.	I know he thinks I am useless. If I say no he will sack me.	Turn that critical voice round; perhaps write it down and test for evidence or assumptions?
Labelling	Using labels or global ratings to describe others or themselves, rather than specific skills or behaviours.	That ward think I'm useless.	If a friend or colleague said something similar, what would you say to them?

Figure 7.1 (Continued)

Thinking error	Description	Example	Try this?
Discounting the positive	Reframing anything positive as unimportant.	My supervisor is only saying that so I will pass the module and she won't have to assess me again!	Ask yourself what you are feeling positive about? How can you ask for feedback that will help you to achieve your goals?
Mental filter/ Focusing on the negative	Focusing on just one negative and judging everything through this. Only focusing on the negative and not on the positives.	My friend never rings me! We are always arguing!	Sometimes we have misunderstood a situation, for whatever reason – perhaps we are feeling tired or stressed and we mistake our thoughts for facts. Ask yourself what evidence are you are using and what thought might be more helpful?
Demands	Peppering your thoughts with rigid and inflexible thinking such as 'shoulds' and 'musts'; making demands of yourself and others.	I should have predicted that was going to happen. He must have known how much that would hurt!	Self-monitoring our thought processes needs daily attention and is helped by writing them down. Being kind and compassionate to yourself is likely to help you regulate demands and reminding yourself you have a choice over what you think can be incredibly liberating!

Figure 7.1 (Continued)

Thinking error	Description	Example	Try this?
Fortune telling/ Catastro-phising	We predict the worst-case scenario	I knew this was going to happen, no one is coming to help, everyone has forgotten. I am going to forget everything – I may as well just go home now!	Using the tool TFA may help you to unpick not just unhelpful thoughts but assumptions too – challenge yourself to identify more helpful thoughts and underpin with evidenced based assumptions? Planning what you need to think and do if the worst happens is good for contingency planning and often helps you to be realistic about what might happen in an emergency.
Low frust-ration tolerance levels or I can't stand it	We lower our tolerance to frustrating or stressful situations by telling ourselves that we can't stand it.	I am not putting up with this anymore!	Perhaps find some middle ground? Ask yourself what might be a more helpful thought in this situation?
Phone-yism	Believing you will get found out by someone important to you as a phoney or imposter.	If I perform badly, they will see the real me – a total fraud!	Find out using feedback what people really feel about what you are doing? Check your assumptions and think about what your positives include?
Blame	Not taking responsibility and blaming somebody or something else for the problem. Abdicating responsibility.	It's their entire fault, they should have recruited an extra person – I can't do it anymore!	Write a list of all the aspects involved in this situation clarify what you can and can't take responsibility for? Invariably health situa-tions are complex issues. Remember we are all human and mainly we try to do our best?

Figure 7.1 Commonly used thinking errors. *Source*: Based on Palmer and Whybrow (2008).

Re-Phrasing

Positivity in language helps us stay focused on the language of change. If we keep on talking about the difficulties or challenges in teaching and learning, our brains remain focused on those difficulties rather than possible solutions. To move our thinking and creativity to solutions we need to use positive language. Using positive language shifts our thinking which in turn releases creativity. The more you insist on something being done, the more resistance you may encounter. As Rogers (2012, p. 40) has argued:

> The best way to change behavior is not to work on what is wrong but to develop new behaviours, creating new neural pathways, which can over a period of time, become dominant.

Mindfulness and relaxation are said to be excellent tools to encourage neuroplasticity, which in simplistic terms helps you to make space in your brain for new ways of doing things.

 Below is an exemplar of a coaching conversation using 'clean' language:

Narrative theory – story telling coaching	Coaching dialogue
Open questioning enables self-reflection.	**Student:** *I don't know what to do.* **Coach**: *And what kind of 'don't know' is don't know?* **Student:** *I'm stuck.* **Coach:** *And is there anything else about 'don't know'?* **Student:** *I feel so useless.*
	Coach: *What happens next?*
Metaphor.	**Student:** *I can't bear it.* **Coach:** *And then what happens?* **Student:** *I let myself down and avoid doing anything!* **Coach:** *And where does that come from?*

Narrative theory – story telling coaching	Coaching dialogue
Rephrasing.	**Student:** *It comes from a feeling I have.* **Coach:** *And where does that feeling come from?* **Student:** *It comes from me thinking I don't know anything!* **Coach:** *And what would be more helpful thinking?* **Student:** *I will have a go at doing something and find out what I need to know!*

The Learning Journey

One of the major challenges of CLiP has been the principle of 'stepping up and stepping back', balancing the adoption of a coaching approach to practice learning whilst ensuring patient safety – giving students more control and autonomy over their learning and practice on the one hand and on the other hand, as supervisors, having to bear the regulatory responsibility and accountability for student learning and patient safety. Thus, of significant importance for supervisors is the ability to not only make competent and confident judgements on the proficiency of students, but also to be able to identify where they are at in their learning journey in order to offer the right level of support to their stage of learning. By learning journey, we mean the journey students are on to be proficient practitioners, i.e. where they are in the process of acquiring knowledge, skills, and attitude in relation to their current placement.

As supervisors, we need to make judgements of students for several reasons:

- To be able to assess their competence to deliver care autonomously and safely for the shift/day that we are supervising.
- To be able to assess the level of support they need, aiming to match their level of need with the right level of support.

- To be able to give feedback contemporaneously to enhance development, i.e. give specific and constructive feedback in the moment or as soon as possible after the performance.
- To be able to articulate and evidence their achievement and contribute to their practice assessments.

There are many tools that can be used to assess where a student is in their learning journey. A common framework used in nursing and midwifery has been Benner's (1984) seminal work on skill acquisition, but it is also worth considering the psychological perspective on the four stages of competence. The work by the American training organisation Gordon Training International in the 1970s and their four stages of competence in Bird and Gornall (2016: p. 85) depicts the learning journey where we move from what the two authors describe as 'blissful ignorance' to 'mastery'. This journey has implications for how our students feel and the way we respond as supervisors.

The unconsciously incompetent learner is day 1 for a student when the size of the task of learning has not yet been communicated or understood, resulting in what we could call blissful ignorance. At this stage students need clear rules, specific guidance, and direction. As a supervisor your role at this stage is very much one of reassurance and even creating a sense of anticipation or excitement of learning journey to come! Promising the learners that they are fully involved and supported in this stage of the journey.

Conscious incompetence is where the learner becomes aware of the size of the task. The student may feel totally overwhelmed by the expectations made of them and the amount of learning seems terrifyingly large. Your role as supervisor here is crucial to the student. Regular check ins and encouragement of students to ask any question they want without fear of ridicule; encouragement of peer-to-peer and team coaching is recommended. Supervisors may support students using the TFA approach as so many of us at this stage of learning feel imposters or discount any positive feedback.

Conscious competence is the third stage of learning. Having learnt a series of new skills, students may feel self-conscious or clumsy in their use of that skill. Students may be aware of high levels of copying their supervisors and colleagues until it becomes an automatic skill. Supervisors need to provide lots of reassurance and positive encouragement at this stage to help the student maintain good practice and make it more natural. Focusing on finding out what they enjoy about their new set of skills helps to reinforce and maintain the student learning.

The last stage is the fourth one of unconscious competence. This is where students do not even notice they are undertaking a particular skill or task because it feels like second nature. There is little need to consult protocols and guidelines because they are all so comfortably used every day. In fact, students may start to coach and supervise others. Building on their knowledge base as well keeps them active in reviewing their actions to avoid complacency.

Figure 7.2 is a framework for facilitating learning that we have adapted from the Blanchard et al. (1985) situational leadership model, integrating the four stages of competence to reflect the stages of the student's learning journey. Each box highlights the behaviour the student might demonstrate and the facilitative behaviour by the coach to support learning.

We have used this framework to demonstrate how we assess, articulate, and evidence the student's learning needs in relation to the level of support provided.

Having Difficult Conversations

Failure to fail has been a major issue in nursing and midwifery students since it was identified in the seminal work by Duffy (2003) – as is supporting failing students. From our experience, the main issues are around adequate and accurate assessment of student competence and feedback. Alongside this we found that mentors were tardy in failing students and they avoided having difficult conversations early on in the placement. Conflict is often part of any collaborative practice and therefore it is important for us all to improve our skills in managing it. There are many positive outcomes to conflict and in brief it is caused by difference – there is an acceptance we need difference for all sorts of sound reasons but the reality of it may frighten us.

Supervision and coaching may result in change or conflict and resisting change sits within us all. Some people find change harder than others. As a supervisor it is our job to help the student uncover what it is they are finding challenging, and doing that demands a high level of trust and

Supportive style	Coaching style
Student demonstrates • Conscious competence • Independent, makes judgements • Range of practice experience • Can explain ideas, apply knowledge to new situations, analyse, and begin to evaluate new ideas **Coach delivers** • Structure • Supervision – indirect supervision, occasional direction • Control – gives responsibility and clear authority	**Student demonstrates** • Conscious incompetence, low/some competence • Counter dependence, averse to seeking help, afraid of showing what they don't know • Some practice experience • Can explain and deliver care, beginning to analyse **Coach delivers** • Structure – clear direction, checks student knows what, why, how • Supervision – moderate level of direct involvement • Control – solicits solutions to solve problems/make decisions • High praise, encourages learning through mistakes/failure
Empowering style	**Directive style**
Student demonstrates • Unconscious competence • Interdependence can be depended on • Intuition • Evaluate and create new knowledge **Coach delivers** • Structure – open to learning from student • Supervision – student may supervise others, indirect supervision • Control – delegates responsibility and authority	**Student demonstrates** • Unconscious incompetence, low competence • Novice, dependent, needs rules • No/limited practice experience • Can define, discuss, and begin to deliver basic care **Coach delivers** • Structure – high level of supervision and attention. Clear information about what, why, and how. Coach needs to validate student has heard the message/instruction • Supervision – commits high amount of time • Control – clear boundaries, structure and regulation

Figure 7.2 Framework for facilitating learning. *Source*: Adapted from Blanchard (1985).

openness. Offering emotional intelligence training to enable clinicians to be more aware of their emotions, and those of their students, might be a way to successful conflict resolution for some.

Before we consider what steps we might take to manage conflict, it is important to review the current skills we are building on. Brockbank and McGill (2013: p. 113) argue that there are three essential skills required by the coach in order to offer the necessary aspect of challenge to coaching conversations – advanced empathy, courage, and existing good relationship.

- *Advanced empathy.* For some supervisors this is tempered by a desire for the student to be similar to himself or herself. The reality, of course, is that everyone is different, and rates of learning and levels of confidence vary dramatically. So, at the heart of this form of empathy lies a degree of humility and genuine curiosity in finding out more about how best to support the learners and individual perception.
  In order to achieve advanced empathy we need to reflectively listen, which is more than just remembering what has been said. Getting a real insight into another person's perspective takes time. Helping the individual untangle feelings from facts maybe a challenge.
- *Courage to confront properly.* It is always hard and takes courage to challenge, especially when you have been working with someone for a while as it is inevitably harder. However, for the student's benefit, it is worth remembering that it is not personal and that it is their behaviours and/or ideas that are being challenged. Using a technique that maintains an effective learning relationship but sometimes moves out of the comfort zone for the student may heighten learning.
- *A good relationship with the person being challenged.* It is important to remember that a neutral adult-to-adult learning style is one that is likely to increase collaboration. With collaboration comes the prospect of greater creativity and confidence in applying new ideas.

Mediation steps include:

1. Understand the issue from both sides.
2. Confront the issue.
3. Define the difficulty.
4. Search for solutions together.
5. Agree on a plan with practical milestones.

References

Benner, P. (1984). From novice to expert, excellence and power in clinical nursing practice. *American Journal of Nursing* 1982: 402–407.

Bird, J. and Gornall, S. (2016). *The Art of Coaching: A Handbook of Tips and Tools*. Abingdon: Routledge.

Blanchard, K.H., Zigarmi, P., and Zigarmi, D. (1985). *Leadership and the One Minute Manager: Increasing Effectiveness through Situational Leadership*. New York: Morrow.

Brockbank, A. and McGill, I. (2013). *Coaching with Empathy*. Maidenhead: McGraw-Hill.

Duffy, K. (2003). *Failing students: A qualitative study of factors that influence the decisions regarding the assessment of students' competence in practice*. http://science.ulster.ac.uk/nursing/mentorship/docs/nursing/oct11/failingstudents.pdf (accessed 2 December 2020).

Palmer and Whybrow (2008). *Handbook of Coaching Psychology*. London/New York: Routledge.

Rogers, J. (2012). *Coaching Skills - a Handbook*, 3e. Maidenhead: Open University Press.

Rogers, J., Whittleworth, K., and Gilbert, A. (2012). *Manager as Coach*. Maidenhead: McGraw-Hill.

Sullivan, W. and Rees, J. (2008). *Clean Language: Revealing Metaphors and Opening Minds*. Camarthan: Crown House Publishing.

Whitmore, J. (2009). *Coaching for Performance: GROWing human potential and purpose*, 4e. London: Brealey.

8

'A Coaching Day'

Rachel Paul, Charlene Lobo and Jonty Kenward

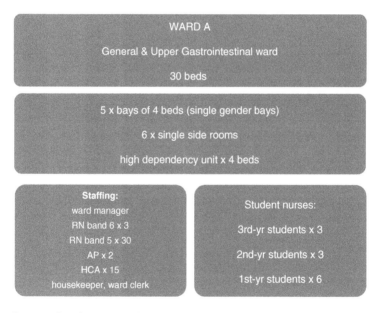

WARD A

General & Upper Gastrointestinal ward

30 beds

5 x bays of 4 beds (single gender bays)

6 x single side rooms

high dependency unit x 4 beds

Staffing:
ward manager
RN band 6 x 3
RN band 5 x 30
AP x 2
HCA x 15
housekeeper, ward clerk

Student nurses:

3rd-yr students x 3

2nd-yr students x 3

1st-yr students x 6

The ward takes general surgery and upper gastrointestinal (GI) carcinomas, colo-rectal surgery and palliative care, namely cardio oesophagectomies, all upper GI stomas, urostomies; high dependency unit (HDU) takes patients post intensive care unit (ICU), which has a specialist nurse managing the unit with a healthcare assistant (HCA) and have a 2 : 1 staff/patient ratio.

Collaborative Learning in Practice: Coaching to Support Student Learners in Healthcare,
First Edition. Charlene Lobo, Rachel Paul, and Kenda Crozier.
© 2021 John Wiley & Sons Ltd. Published 2021 by John Wiley & Sons Ltd.
Companion website: www.wiley.com/go/lobo/collaborativelearninginpractice

Per shift, the ward is staffed as follows: one registered nurse (RN) in charge, three other RNs and three HCAs per 12-hour day shift to care for the patients on the ward. In addition, there is a ward manager who works Monday to Friday and sometimes works clinically. Staffing is reduced to four on a night shift. The staff are organised into two teams that each look after half the ward, i.e. 19 patients.

There is a CLiP™ lead for the a Trust, and an educational team that comprises one senior management registered nurse (known as Band 7 in the UK), 4 senior clinical registered nurses (known as Band 6 in the UK), and 3 assistant practitioners plus admin, who do the training on the ward for CLiP and support the supervisors on the ward. Each ward has learning environment managers who are nominated to student coordination protected time each week to undertake student induction, off-duty, and to support student learning in the ward environment.

This case study is based on a fictitious day in the life of a coach. We have focused on some of key points where there might be conversations between coach and students. Of course there will be many conversations, individually and collectively, that are not carried out in such depth; but in these scenarios we have aimed to demonstrate the key principles of coaching, use some of our basic theoretical frameworks for conversation and, most importantly, articulate facilitation of learning in the language of coaching.

Mabelline is the coach for ward A today. She is responsible for the care of 10 patients in two bays and two side rooms. She has HCA Gaby and student nurses Olatu, Joe, Gemma, and Rachel working with her today.

Bay 1:	Bay 2:
2 patients for surgery	1 for surgery
1 patient 3rd day post-op	2 patients self-caring post-operatively
1 patient for discharge	1 patient for discharge
	1 admission

Side room 1	Side room 2
Mr X is six days post surgery following an intended cardio-oesophagectomy. The outcome was not as expected as they were unable to remove the tumour. Mr X moved out of HDU yesterday and is in the process of moving on to palliative care.	Mrs Y has dementia; she had a feeding tube inserted a week ago but has now got MRSA.

Olatu is a third-year student, in her first week of placement on this ward but towards the end of her training, she has not met Mabelline or the others before.

Joe is second year and has been on the ward for four weeks, he is halfway through the second year. He has worked several times with Mabelline before and has also worked with both Gemma and Gaby.

Gemma is a first-year student who has been working on the ward for three weeks; this is her second placement but her first surgical care experience. She hasn't been supervised by Mabelline before but has worked with both Joe and Gaby.

Rachel is a nursing apprentice, it is her first placement and she has been on the ward for two weeks. However, Rachel has worked as a HCA for the past six months on another surgical ward before applying for her nursing apprenticeship.

Gaby is a very experienced healthcare assistant whose role is to contribute to patient care.

Scenario 1: Beginning the Shift, Managing and Negotiating Student-Led Learning

It is 7.30 a.m. on an eight-hour shift and the team have just taken the handover from the night shift.

 Things to think about

Make some notes in answer to the following questions:

- How would you start your day?
- How do you support student-led approaches to learning in the context of care delivery?
- How would you manage competing demands for you to supervise?
- How do you work out each student's learning journey – novice to expert/incompetent competence?
- How will you go about allocating the care of your patients and organising the day?

 Applying Theory to Practice

This scenario is based on the type of conversation to be had at the beginning of the shift with the coach, students, and other members of the team. It involves establishing a relationship, identifying what the students' learning outcomes for the shift are, and establishing where they are in their learning journey. We need to be mindful of the principles of coaching (Chapter 5). If the learning is student led, then the support given is so much more likely to be listened to and acted on. The idea of 'you insist, I resist' is something we mentioned in Chapter 5; it is key to establishing collaborative working. The use of positive and 'clean' language (Chapter 7) is essential in building self-confidence and establishing trusting relationships where students feel able to ask for help. Clearly communicating expectations is an essential part of the process.

 ## Exemplar of a Coaching Conversation

Signposting the theory	Coaching dialogue
Goal focused with some evidence of being student led as each person is encouraged to summarise where they perceive they are at in their different learning journeys. Mabelline is also explicit about her goal, so setting an example that this is a collaborative process where everyone has a goal. Friendly invitation to start them off.	**Mabelline:** *Morning everyone, I am Mabelline and am your coach. My goal for this shift is to ensure I have observed each of you achieve your identified learning outcomes. I don't think I have met all of you before and haven't worked with some of you before. So let's start by introducing ourselves, highlighting where we are at, and identifying what our goals are for this shift. Who wants to start?*
Some justification offered to continue the care of Mr H.	**Joe:** *OK I'll start: I am Joe, I am almost at the end of my second year and halfway through this placement. I was on yesterday and looked after Mr H with the SN so would like to continue with his care today.*
It sounds like Gemma's goal could be to increase familiarity with the patients/placement/patient conditions? Gemma communicated a slight nervousness as she had been off for a couple of days.	**Gemma:** *I am Gemma, first-year student nurse. this is my first placement and I have been on this ward for three weeks and I was off for the last two days so am not familiar with any of the patients.*

Signposting the theory	Coaching dialogue
It is important that Gemma's feelings are acknowledged so that she can start to feel supported and able to voice her feelings and needs. It is also important to get the rest of the students to start acknowledgement and support to build effective working relationships.	**Mabelline:** *Don't worry Gemma you will soon get to know them – they are really lovely. What do the rest of you think?*
Honest and open response from Olatu adds to the feeling of support and openness between them. Clear goal and outcomes stated, but some specific outcomes would be even better.	**Olatu:** *They are very sweet, but some are really poorly. By the way I am Olatu, a third-year student on my final placement, and I want to complete my management outcomes on this ward.*
Mabbelline's recognition of positive support potentially encourages even more support. Being specific about the outcomes will increase the likelihood of them being recognised and hopefully achieved.	**Mabelline:** *Good point Olatu – thanks. Now tell me more about which of the management outcomes you need to focus on today?*
	Olatu: *I think I need to develop my leadership skills in managing others*
	Rachel: *I am Rachel, I am a nurse apprentice and have just started the course but have been on the ward for the last six months. I would like to meet my pre and post-op learning outcomes*
Essential to include the whole team. We are all equal.	**Mabelline:** *And what about you Gaby?*
Gaby communicated how open and flexible she is.	**Gaby:** *I am Gaby, I have worked on this ward for the last five years and I was on shift yesterday and I'm happy to help anyone with patient care. How it normally works is the students need to work out between themselves who needs me to help them first.*

Signposting the theory	Coaching dialogue
Now Mabelline begins to establish the context or reality of expectations for the day, as well as focusing on the needs of patients. In addition she is communicating her expectations of both performance and check-in times. This initial directing is crucial in both motivation and learning, so that students can gain a sense of both what is expected of them and when it will be possible to get support and help.	**Mabelline:** *OK. Thanks Gaby that's great.* *Welcome everyone! We have a busy shift ahead. This is how we will work the day: we will first agree which patients you want to look after, taking into account your individual skills development, learning outcomes, and most importantly balancing it with patient need.*
It's often a balancing act when you have different students with different expectations and learning outcomes to achieve. Clear boundaries creating a safe environment (principle 2).	*Then I will come to each of you and we can discuss how you plan your work and what specific supervision you need; we need to agree on breaks now so that we can make sure we cover for each other. I'd like for us to all catch up midway through the shift, maybe just after lunch, and then I'd like to have time with each of you at the end for feedback. So, I will start with you Joe, you have already identified the patient you want to care for, any other patients?*
When you set a culture of collaboration then hopefully students will start to think for themselves about what they can do and take ownership of responsibilities.	**Joe:** *I could look after some others in one of the bays?*
Important to use open and probing questions that give students a chance to not only to think for themselves but take into account what they have previously communicated in terms of their needs or expectations.	**Mabelline:** *OK; how do you feel about working with Rachel and taking care of patients in bay 2? If you and Rachel make your way there and start with reviewing the care plans, I will catch up with you as soon as I have finished with Olatu and Gemma? So, what about you two what do you want to achieve today*
Energy and motivation clearly communicated.	**Joe:** *Great! Come on Rachel, let's go.*

Signposting the theory	Coaching dialogue
Rachel and Joe both communicate they are feeling positive with a sense of energy for getting things done.	**Rachel:** *OK with me!*
Good sign of open communication when students express what they need. Student sets the agenda (principle 4).	**Olatu:** *Well, I need to do some management.*
Being open about needs makes it so much easier for them to look at how they can meet those needs within the restrictions of ward management.	**Gemma:** *I don't know the patients.*
Again its crucial to encourage students to take ownership as far as possible with what assessment they need to achieve and how they are going to integrate it into the everyday workings of the ward. It is up to Olatu to be familiar with the specific outcomes and for Mabelline to trust Olatu to know them. If they are wildly out of kilter with Mabelline's expectations, then she may just question or check Olatu's source of information or interpretation.	**Mabelline:** *OK, so let's start with you Olatu. What are your specific outcomes for this management unit?*
This sounds quite ambiguous – worth digging a bit deeper?	**Olatu:** *Well, being in charge.*
Good to be clear about the specific longer term outcome as well as the short-term goal.	**Mabelline:** *Being in charge of what specifically?*

Signposting the theory	Coaching dialogue
Great to be this determined!	**Olatu:** *The ward!*
Important to acknowledge the ambition, but Mabelline needs to find out relevant experience in order to be able to support her to achieve this goal. Develop student's resourcefulness (principle 2).	**Mabelline** *Good for you! So, when have you been in charge of a ward before?*
Student describes experience.	**Olatu:** *At the end of my second year I managed a bay, but my last placement was ITU so I mainly did one-to-one nursing*
Mabelline gets some in-depth analysis and evaluation of that experience with open and probing questions in order to gain insight into Olatu's competency level. The student is resourceful and has got previous experience (principle 1).	**Mabelline** *What did it feel like have total accountability and responsibility of a patient's care?*
Positive feedback indicated a great enthusiasm for learning.	**Olatu:** *I got great feedback and absolutely loved doing those things!*
Good to be more specific about the requirements in order to challenge.	**Mabelline:** *Well done! What about managing teams or delegating work?*
Open and honest in response.	**Olatu:** *No I didn't really have much opportunity to do that.*
Good to summarise and at the same time check your understanding and the student's as to what they are comfortable with.	**Mabelline:** *OK Olatu; so just to double check, you have been here for three days and what you are saying is that you are comfortable with the ward routine and the care delivery?*
Positive reflection on previous experiences.	**Olatu:** *Oh yes; I did a previous two-week placement here and asked to come back for my final placement as I would like to work on here when I am qualified.*

Signposting the theory	Coaching dialogue
Motivational opportunity presented to overarching goal with a start in that journey; supporting Gemma and increasing her confidence.	**Mabelline:** *Brilliant – so here's a possible start to being in charge of a ward, how about you and Gemma work together on bay 1 and side room with Mrs Y. I will leave you and Gemma to look over the care plans and I will come back after I've been to see Joe and Rachel.*

 ## Self-Learning

Compare this conversation to the notes you made in the 'think about' section. What are the similarities and the differences? Note how the positive supportive mindset/perspective influences the language and tone of the conversation. Reflecting on the coaching dialogue in the above scenario, what do you think you need to focus on to develop your supervision style to be an even better coach?

 Go to the companion website for examples of how we might assess each student's learning journey.

Scenario 2: One-to-One Supervision – Using a Coaching Approach to Assess/Make Judgements About Student Competence/the Level of Supervision Needed

Following on from the previous conversation, Mabelline has gone to catch up with Joe and Rachel.

 ## Things to Think About

- How will Mabelline work out where each student is on their learning journey?
- How will Mabelline assess each student's competence in order to feel confident that they are able to safely deliver care independently and also work out what level of support each student needs?
- How will Mabelline help students identify the learning outcomes they wish to achieve for the shift?

Applying Theory to Practice

In this scenario, we have used the OSCAR model of coaching and Miller's pyramid of clinical competence in an integrated manner to establish the learning outcome and to also enable the coach to assure themselves of the competence of the student undertaking the task.

Exemplar of a Coaching Conversation

Signposting theory	Coaching dialogue
Open questioning to determine agreed outcome by the two students.	**Mabelline:** *OK Joe and Rachel; how have you decided to split the work between you two?*
Situation clearly described to communicate the context in which the students are working.	**Joe:** *We thought we could have a post-op patient each and as I have Mr X who needs a lot of initial care, Rachel would prepare Mrs A for surgery and then organise the discharge for Mrs C, and I would prepare for the admission.*
	Mabelline: *Does that work for you Rachel in meeting your learning outcomes?*
	Rachel: *Yes, I need to learn how to complete a pre-operative checklist.*
It doesn't really make much difference if you use the headings of OSCAR in a different order. It would also be helpful to the student if you are transparent about any coaching model you are using so that they can use it for themselves with colleagues or to self-coach.	**Mabelline:** *Brilliant Rachel, well organised. So, Joe, besides delivering care to your two patients what specific outcomes or new learning do you want to achieve on this shift?*
Outcomes clearly identified.	**Joe:** *I would like to remove the drain on Mr X; the staff nurse showed me how to do one yesterday.*
Situation – the starting point, what is Joe's knowledge base before he delivers the care?	**Mabelline:** *OK Joe; so explain to me as if I were the patient and this was the first time you were doing my dressing what you are going to do. Remember you need to explain to me about drains.*

Signposting theory	Coaching dialogue
Joe has clearly communicated his knowledge base and is beginning to demonstrate application of knowledge in relation to patient condition	Joe is able to explain competently about Mr X's drain where it sits (A&P), and why Mr X has it.
Mabelline is further probing Joe's knowledge base on the procedure. As Joe begins to explain the procedure, he begins to consider **choices and consequences** – why he is undertaking certain procedures.	**Mabelline:** *That's good Joe; so now how would you explain what is involved in the removing the drain?*
Mabelline is establishing Joe's evidence of knowledge.	Joe is able to clearly explain the procedure, he has intimated that he has also looked it up on clinical skills net.
Recognition will add to Joe's source of motivation and may result in increased energy and motivation to learn more and perform well. **Choice and consequences** – exploring red flag situations. Using open and probing questions to check 'knows how' (Miller's competency framework).	**Mabelline:** *That's really good Joe. I'm also impressed that you looked it up as it shows that you have prepared for today.* *What are the things you are looking out for when you carry out the procedure?* *Tell me more about what might be of concern and anything you would need to report?*
	Joe is able to explain clearly the red flags for removing a drain.
Action – doing it.	**Mabelline:** *Great, looks like you clearly know what you are doing, let's go and do it.*
Review	**Mabelline:** *Well done Joe, how did that feel?*

 ## *Self-Learning*

How does this approach compare to your experiences of helping a student identify a learning outcome? How could you apply this approach to outcomes achievable in your area of practice? Have a go and try to apply this approach to learning outcomes in your area of practice.

Go to the companion website for an example of Joe's learning log to see how his performance was assessed and documented.

Scenario 3: Checking in Midway Conversation

This is a conversation that is conducted with Mabelline and the team halfway through the shift and just after the lunch break. It is an opportunity for Mabelline to check on patient safety and student safety. From a patient safety perspective, it means checking the patient condition (interrogating the evidence by questioning the student/patient/recorded observations) as well as making sure all required care has been delivered to a satisfactory standard. From a student safety perspective, checking to make sure students are feeling confident in their care delivery, ensuring they are on target to meet outcomes, and ensuring that they are receiving the right facilitation for their learning.

 ### *Things to Think About*

- Where do you think the students are on their learning journeys?
- How would you evaluate the supervisor support offered in meeting the needs of the students?
- How would you encourage students to maximise the use of learning resources available and to check on themselves and support each other?
- How will you as a student or as a supervisor update outcomes for learning and any identified gaps?

 ### *Applying Theory to Practice*

Checking students' performance isn't coaching and this paradox is something we have looked at before. Assessment is about passing judgement, and coaching is about withholding judgement. However, we can still make use of coaching skills and approaches both as a supervisor and as a student to help achieve the expected performance. As a supervisor you need to be transparent about when you are assessing and when you are coaching. Keeping track of student progress is important for both the student and patient, encouraging the student to regularly check medication and the application of safe patient care. The example below aims to demonstrate how coaching approaches have been used in the informal assessment of student performance.

 ### Exemplar of a coaching conversation – catching up with all the team, challenging students to extend their learning

Signposting theory	Coaching dialogue
Mabelline's opening question demonstrates a commitment to equality (principle 5) the student sets the agenda (principle 4).	**Mabelline:** *OK. Let's check-in with where we are all at. Who wants to start?*
Joe is very positive reflecting the student is resourceful (principle 1). When there is a positive response, this can indicate increased confidence and this is helpful for further challenge and learning.	**Joe:** *We will. We're up-to-date with all our work. I'm really pleased I managed to take Mr X's drain and am waiting for feedback on that.*
Mabelline setting realistic expectations with students in an adult-to-adult communication (principle 1). Clear boundary setting (principle 2).	**Mabelline:** *That's good Joe, I will give you more in-depth written feedback at the end of the shift but at present I just want to make sure we have caught up with all the care and I am checking on how the patients are doing … and Rachel?*
Descriptive list offered only.	**Rachel:** *Mrs A has gone to theatre, Mrs C is waiting for the pharmacist to see her before she goes home, but I'm not sure about Mrs B.*
More powerful open question used to elicit more information.	**Mabelline:** *OK, so tell me more about Mrs B?*
	Rachel: *Well her temp was up at 10.00 so as you know I told the doctor and he ordered some bloods to be done. The patient is still waiting for this but in the meantime I gave them paracetamol.*

Signposting theory	Coaching dialogue
The coach's role is to develop the student's resourcefulness through skilful questioning, challenge (principle 2). This 'what else' question is always a simple but useful form of challenge.	**Mabelline:** *That's really good. What else could you do to make the patient more comfortable?*
Rachel is using her open questioning skills with colleagues to help find out more about their experiences in order to collaborate in their work with patients.	**Rachel:** *Gaby, you've been working with Mrs B, what else could we do?*
Gaby was encouraged to offer her experience and ideas, the collaboration results in something else to consider.	**Gaby:** *Well although I'm not completely sure, in my experience some patients with high temperatures have an infection?*
Helping Gaby build her resourcefulness (principle 1) encouraging Gaby to set her own agenda about how she fills her knowledge gap	**Mabelline:** *When have you come across a patient who has presented with a high temp before?*
Helping Rachel recognise she has past knowledge and believes in herself enhances motivation and self-confidence (principle 1, 2, 3).	**Rachel:** *A couple of times when they have had an infection. I think I need to focus a bit on Mrs B and consider what other options I might use to reduce her temp.*
Supervisor is interpreting Rachel response as a commitment to relevant research. More directing than coaching.	**Mabelline:** *That sounds like a perfect subject for you to pursue in your research hour, let me know how you get on.*
Open question, but very general and not challenging.	**Mabelline:** *OK; Olatu and Gemma where are you at?* **Olatu:** *We're good, all up-to-date.*
Questions need to be specific to draw specific answers.	
Try and avoid multiple questions – both these questions are potentially big so give lots of space and time to answer or ask one question at a time?	**Mabelline:** *OK, more specifically what do you feel is going on in terms of your patients' conditions and how do you feel about the care you have delivered so far?*

Signposting theory	Coaching dialogue
Very descriptive summary, no sense of any learning gained.	**Olatu:** *I think we are up-to-date. We've got one dressing to do this afternoon and Mrs Y is waiting for her scan this afternoon and Gemma will go with her to see the procedure.*
This is the result of Olatu's directive style – a passive and differential child response. Gemma is looking at Olatu to have all the answers and do all the work and thus reducing her own confidence.	**Gemma:** *It was nice working with Olatu, she explained everything to me. I don't know how she remembered all the things we had to do for all the patients.*
Olatu enjoying her status, adoration, compliments.	**Olatu:** *Well it comes with practice.*
Evidence that Olatu has squashed Gemma's confidence, not giving Gemma opportunities.	**Gemma:** *Yeah but it really scares me as I feel I will miss something and remembering so many patients.*
Supervisor building students by support (principle 2) recognition that Gemma needs to believe in herself.	**Mabelline:** *Well Gemma, I suppose it begins with one patient and builds from there. How have you delivered patient care today?*
Clear evidence of the impact of using a directing approach, implying Gemma has spent the day following Olatu but not developing herself or her confidence.	**Gemma:** *I've been working with Olatu, she's mainly told me what to do and when to do it.*
Supportive questioning and reflective listening to draw out Gemma's insights.	**Mabelline:** *And how has that that make you feel?*
This is the cost to Gemma of being directed all day.	**Gemma:** *At the time I found it reassuring and helpful to be told what to do, but now I feel a bit useless and that I don't know anything.*
The coaching conversation is all about looking forward and finding even better ways of working together.	**Mabelline:** *OK Olatu, so having listened to Gemma and how she feels now, how might you adapt your management style in supporting Gemma?*

Signposting theory	Coaching dialogue
Olatu has moved from a parent to child relationship to an adult-to-adult (principle 5). Olatu believes in Gemma, that she is resourceful, communicating that she has trust in her and therefore she is more likely to believe it in herself (principle 2). It hasn't become too much of a habit to break out from being directed, and despite the nervousness there is a sense of excitement in taking on more responsibility.	**Olatu:** *I think I missed the point here, I haven't applied any coaching skills. So maybe this afternoon Gemma, you and I can work together where you take the lead and I support you. How do you feel about taking charge of Mr A and Mr B? I completely trust you to manage this and you know where to get help if you need it.* **Gemma:** *I feel a bit nervous but I would really like to take on that responsibility.*

Self-Learning

From the above conversations and using the learning facilitation model, where do you think Joe and Olatu were in their learning journeys?

 Go to the companion website to see how Olatu's performance has been documented in her learning log.

Scenario 4: End of a Shift – Using Coaching Approaches to Giving Feedback

It is nearing the end of the shift and Mabelline has to give feedback to the students orally as well as fill in their learning logs to supply the written evidence of achievement. This scenario will focus on Gemma and Olatu.

Things to Think About

- What feedback would you be giving students?
- As a supervisor, how would you be assessing them?
- How would you evidence this in their paperwork?

Applying Theory to Practice

Always remember that feedback is two-way. The feedback you give communicates your priorities, observations, and a lot of information about what you value as well as what your student observes, prioritises, and values! If done constructively, feedback is a great trigger for change and action! To find better ways of thinking about things, and therefore feeling differently, which may ultimately lead to different actions – feedback can be powerful! Regular reviews and de-briefs potentially give learners an opportunity to clarify their learning and review their progress in achieving learning or professional development goals.

On the other hand, feedback can be just an excuse to tell people what you think they should be doing. Thereby losing the opportunity for students to learn, develop new skills and confidence. It is important to agree with your students how and when you will give them feedback as well as asking for feedback on your coaching with them. It reminds them that this is a collaborative process, where learning is a continuous process, regardless of expertise, and also demonstrates your commitment to an egalitarian culture.

In this particular scenario, although all students have done well in achieving their objective there is always opportunity to learn more and as a coach the job is to push and challenge more. For Olatu, there is opportunity as a third-year student to coach Gemma and assess and give feedback on her practice; and for Gemma, she could have explored the concept of total patient care.

 ## Exemplar of a Coaching Conversation Giving Feedback

This exemplar conversation is had between Mabelline, Olatu, and Gemma.

Signposting the theory	Coaching dialogue
Positive mindset from the start helped to create a positive environment for discussion and learning.	**Mabelline:** *OK you have excellent feedback from John. The patients in Bay 2, they say they feel well cared for. How do you both feel about that?*
Further positive reinforcement.	**Olatu:** *That's great, they're really good patients.*

Signposting the theory	Coaching dialogue
Completion of tasks.	**Gemma:** *We had a really good plan and we achieved everything on it!*
Now we start to uncover what they felt they enjoyed. Learning theory – learning through 'joyful stress'.	**Mabelline:** *That's great! What was it that you feel you enjoyed the most?*
Adults are more interested in solving real-life problems, motivated by an internal sense of purpose.	**Gemma:** *For me it was working with Olatu, it helped me feel more confident we were able to be efficient in solving problems together. Olatu has taught me a lot.*
Reflecting a similar mindset and commitment to making a difference will have encouraged a sense of collaboration.	**Olatu:** *I agree – having someone else to share the tasks and responsibility made everything so much easier! So much faster!*
Recognition of what they have enjoyed is crucial to stimulating the student's intrinsic sense of motivation, offering a clear challenge.	**Mabelline:** *That's great teamwork then! Having been able to work more efficiently together and achieve the outcomes required, what is your next challenge?*
Extending what students have already seen to be the primary issue to wider needs.	**Gemma:** *I think I need to learn more about how to manage the care of a patient on my own?*
Clear expression of an area of interest makes for a good start.	**Olatu:** *I don't think I know enough about managing and coaching a team?*
Encouraging a mindset of openness and capability of change with positive feedback and encouragement.	**Mabelline:** *It's great you are both so positive and committed to following up on those specific areas of learning.*
Meeting the needs of the assessment requirements is crucial and relevant forms are carefully completed to provide specific evidence of criteria achieved or not yet achieved plus questioning used to check knowledge and understanding.	*First things first, however; we need to complete your learning logs before looking forward to the next as the skills you have developed will be of great use in going forward to developing yourselves even further.*
The supervisor goes into a neutral role and one that can focus on the feedback process encouraging Olatu now to step up as coach. The offer of help is genuinely communicated.	*We need to look now at the specific skills you have demonstrated and give each other both some peer feedback and coaching. What do you need from me to help you?*

Signposting the theory	Coaching dialogue
Olatu assumes a supervisor role comfortably, appearing confident and collaborative.	**Olatu:** *We thought you would ask us that, so we completed feedback on each other in writing and we would like you to observe us giving that feedback to each other. We have started to fill in the learning logs.*
The reality is that most people need time to work out the details of their development plan.	**Mabelline:** *That's an excellent start! Let's look at these together.*

Self-Learning

Based on the above conversation, how might this influence the feedback form you fill in the learning logs? Have a go at filling in a learning log for Joe and Rachel.

9

Acute Adult Care – Orthopaedic and Trauma Ward

Rachel Paul, Charlene Lobo and Helen Bell

> **Adult Orthopaedic and Trauma**
>
> **38 beds**

> **4 x bays of 6 beds (single gender)**
>
> **and 12 x single side rooms**

> Student nurses:
> 4 x 1st-years-first placement/6 (Dion, Josie, Paris and Georgia) 2 x 4 week blocks of placements
> separated by 5 weeks in school
> 2 x 2nd-years-fourth placement/6 (Anna and Niramon) 9-week block of placement
> 2 x 3rd-years fifth placement/6 (Lola and Kamran) 10-week block of placement
> 1 x trainee nursing associate (2-year apprenticeship) (Chloe) -first year, home ward
> Total = 9

The ward is staffed as follows: one registered nurse (RN) in charge, three other RNs and three healthcare assistants (HCA) per 12-hour day shift to care for the patients on the ward. In addition, there is a ward manager who works Monday to Friday and sometimes works clinically. Staffing is reduced to four on a night shift. The staff are organised into two teams that each look after half the ward, i.e. 19 patients.

A clinical educator, George, supports student nurses (direct entry and Nursing Degree Apprentices [NDAs]), new members of staff and other learners, e.g. overseas nurses, return to practice, HCAs, trainee nursing

Collaborative Learning in Practice: Coaching to Support Student Learners in Healthcare, First Edition. Charlene Lobo, Rachel Paul, and Kenda Crozier.
© 2021 John Wiley & Sons Ltd. Published 2021 by John Wiley & Sons Ltd.
Companion website: www.wiley.com/go/lobo/collaborativelearninginpractice

associates (TNAs), and is the 'nominated person' for the ward. The clinical educator is part of a practice education and development team that supports clinical areas across the hospital. George is an experienced clinical educator having four years' experience in the role and has facilitated and supported the development of several clinical wards that have adopted a contemporary collaborative model of learning. George has worked with the deputy sister, who is the ward's education lead for learners, to plan the students off-duty, including a rotation of multidisciplinary spoke placements to other areas such as: clean elective orthopaedic ward, pre-assessment clinic, theatres and recovery, physiotherapy, occupational therapy, fracture clinic, radiology, hip and knee school, pain team, outpatients department, orthopaedic pharmacy, and the orthopaedic nurse practitioner team. Students and staff usually work 12.5-hour day and night shifts (07.00–19.30 or 19.00–07.30) but shorter early and late shifts are also available (07.00–13.00 or 13.00–19.30). Students work in the same team as their practice supervisor but not necessarily their practice assessor.

Kamran is a third-year student nurse who is undertaking his fifth and penultimate clinical placement; the learning outcomes for this module of learning focus on the care of adult patients with acute complex needs. He has previously undertaken a range of clinical placements in a community nursing team, a cardiology ward, ENT outpatients and a rehabilitation ward in a community hospital. He is now in the fourth week of his 10-week placement and feels confident that he is progressing very well. He feels supported by the staff that have offered a variety of learning opportunities and worked with him quite closely. To date, Kamran has achieved good marks in all theoretical assignments with marks of over 60% using minimal support from his personal academic advisor, and all assignments have been passed at first attempt. He has also passed all his previous practice related assessments with mostly positive comments from mentors (prior to NMC Standards for Student Supervision and Assessment – SSSA) and subsequently practice supervisors/assessors on his last placement.

Anna is a second-year student nurse and is in the last two weeks of placement on this ward. Previously, she has successfully completed a variety of community- and hospital-based clinical placements and has passed all theoretical assignments to date with good marks. She has become quite confident on the ward and has led the care of six patients, delegating tasks to HCAs and a first-year student nurse as required. She feels that she has developed a good relationship with most of the staff on the ward, particularly the HCAs and her practice supervisor, Issy; however, Anna has found it difficult to discuss her learning and clinical issues with Sam, her practice assessor, who is one of two deputy sisters on the ward. Anna feels that Sam can sometimes be judgemental towards certain groups of patients, such as substance misusers, that she doesn't give enough attention to providing individualised care for patients and that she prefers to spend more time with the doctors.

Scenario 1: A Positive Perspective of the 'Failing Student': Helping Students Understand Their Development Needs and Action Planning to Meet Them

Kamran's practice assessor, Rachel, has asked for a meeting with him and the link lecturer to discuss his progression, prior to his formative assessment next week (mid-point), as she wants to raise some negative feedback from the medical team and also some concerning issues when calculating drug dosages.

 Things to Think About

- Kamran appears very confident, although on closer inspection, is not meeting learning outcomes.
- It seems from discussion that previous mentors/supervisors have not challenged his practical skills in Year 1 and 2.
- From a coaching perspective, we would propose there is no such thing as a 'failing student' and to consider a more empowering concept. How could the situation be re-framed?
- What is it like to feel part of a team that have mutual respect even if you make an error?
- Staff negotiated a very detailed action plan with Kamran that clearly showed how he could achieve his goals, i.e. who he would work with each shift, and specific learning tasks he would be set according to the way he would find useful.

Applying Theory to Practice

'Students at risk of failing' or 'failing students' are terms commonly used in describing student performance that is not on track or meeting identified outcomes. From a coaching perspective, it is a disempowering concept and one we feel is contradictory to coaching philosophy. From our perspective, we have re-framed the concept as understanding and helping students understand their development needs.

- Adult-to-adult rapport is encouraged to achieve ownership of any development needed.
- Core skills of coaching used are open questioning and reflective listening out for emotions that help to pick up on the back-story.
- Clinical educators provide a fresh face and new perspective to resolving tricky problems.
- The unwilling coachee has a back-story, which is often hard to understand for complex reasons.

 ## Exemplar of a Coaching Conversation

Signposting theory	Coaching conversation
Rationale provided for conversation. Adult-to-adult interaction clarified.	**Rachel:** *This is a good time to discuss progress and expectations before your mid-point formative assessment. It's a opportunity to provide you with some feedback and discuss your progression so far. How do you feel that your placement is going?*
Good open question to extract much needed perception on progress with emphasis on feelings.	
Some balanced but positive reflection offered.	**Kamran:** *I think the placement is going really well and I feel confident. I'm happy to take the lead on a group of patients' care and I think I've been doing a good job. I don't think that I want to work here when I qualify though.*

Signposting theory	Coaching conversation
Reflective listening to build rapport so that the student can think more for himself about what has led him to the conclusion he wouldn't want to work on that ward again.	**Rachel:** *That's interesting feedback Kamran. Tell me more about what has made you decide that?*
Kamran quickly opens up to the issue of calculating IV drug doses and the difference of opinion with his qualified and experienced colleague.	**Kamran:** *One of the nurses said that I was calculating an IV drug dose incorrectly, but I disagreed with her and still think that my answer was correct. She just didn't like the way that I calculated it, as it was different to her way. She doesn't like me because I'm quite confident.*
Rachel shows Kamran written feedback that the nurse drawing up the IV drugs had repeatedly shown Kamran why his calculations were incorrect but that he had refused to accept that he was wrong. This had occurred on two or three separate occasions with two different RNs. He had argued with the supervising nurse.	**Rachel:** *Kamran can I give you some feedback?* (Kamran nods in agreement.) **Rachel:** *Let's look at the written notes from your colleagues?* **Kamran:** *OK.* **Rachel:** *How about having a chat with George our clinical educator – he is happy to support you too.*
By introducing George as another supporter there is a chance that a different perspective will help clear the air and help Kamran move forward.	**George:** *Thanks for agreeing to see me Kamran.* **Kamran:** *No problem.*
Highlight the danger to the patient and lack of respect shown to the supervising nurse. Further discussion about the rationale for having two checkers and how you would respond as a qualified nurse if you both calculate a different result – mutual respect, checking each other's calculations, and resolving the issue in a professional manner.	**George:** *What evidence were you using that made you so sure that you were correct on those calculations, ignoring your qualified colleagues who have lots of experience?*

Signposting theory	Coaching conversation
Kamran felt sure he was right because he hasn't been picked up on anything before in a placement and has very high marks for assignments.	**Kamran:** *I have never been told before that I was wrong using this same approach!* **George:** *Never?* **Kamran:** *All that was given to me were development plans!* **George:** *What do you believe was the purpose of those development plans?*
Kamran is resistant to this negative feedback saying that those nurses don't like him, possibly because he is very confident, he doesn't know why they feel that way. Rachel also feeds back that the medical team and some members of staff have found him abrupt. Reflectively listening to uncover the backstory. Checking assumptions. Getting buy-in from Kamran. Checking the facts. Maybe a misunderstanding of the purpose of the plans Clarification of the purpose of the plans.	**Kamran:** *Some of the nurses here don't like me! I didn't realise I was doing those calculations the wrong way!* *I don't know what they mean by being abrupt?* **George:** *You sound really upset Kamran. Let me just check I have understood you correctly?* **Kamran:** OK. **George:** *No one has corrected your calculations?* **Kamran:** *They just gave me development plans.* **George:** *OK Kamran, that is the process for supporting you to develop your skills further in response to mistakes with your calculations.*
Surprise – little self-awareness. Building rapport to support a positive outcome. Great use of powerful open questions to extract Kamran's interpretation maintaining a student-led approach. Kamran offering more data about his situation and his feelings. Encourages Kamran to reflect on how he feels he comes across to others. Good self-realisation. More challenging question to trigger deeper reflection. Kamran communicates his approach.	**Kamran:** *Really?* **George:** *Yes. Sorry you were not made aware of that.* **Kamran:** *What about being abrupt?* **George:** *What do you think that means?* **Kamran:** *I don't know? I have lots to fit in to my day and I have a lot going on in my life so I can get frustrated sometimes.* **George:** *How do you express that frustration?* **Kamran:** *I get to the point quickly.* **George:** *What reaction do you get in return?*

Signposting theory	Coaching conversation
George encourages Kamran to start reflecting on the impact of his behaviour. More information on how Kamran is feeling. George respectfully checks that he can offer feedback before giving it thereby increasing the acceptance of it.	**Kamran**: *I don't really wait around as I have to get on.* **George:** *So, what is the impact on your colleagues if they perceive you are keen to get on?* **Kamran:** *I didn't think they noticed me or even cared.* **George:** *OK Kamran can I give you some feedback?* **Kamran:** *OK.*
George communicated a positive message that Kamran will take away and reflect on further. Remember we are all humans trying to do our best, and real change only happens in baby steps.	**George:** *The fact that they have given you development plans demonstrates they want you to grow and achieve your potential. The feedback about being abrupt is also further evidence that they want to interact with you but feel you are reluctant to?* *I want you to meet the link lecturer and work out where you go from here.*
An action plan is formed and agreed with the practice supervisor.	Kamran reluctantly agrees to working out a skills development plan that will help him succeed.

Self-Learning

Supervisor
- How would you feel in this situation?
- What would you do to help Kamran reflect on the outcome he needs to succeed?
- How will you encourage a coaching culture in your practice?
- What further reading/learning do you need to do to enhance your practice?

Student
- What could you do if this happened to you?
- Where would you go for support?
- How would you feel in this situation?
- What might you say to a peer in a similar situation?

Scenario 2: 'There is no such thing as a failing student'

Second Meeting Between Kamran and the LL in the School

The link lecturer (LL) meets separately with Kamran in the school later that week at the student's request. The student continues to insist that he has done nothing wrong. The LL has verified that the student has indeed done very well in assignments and passed previous placements. The LL made it clear to Kamran that he would not pass his assessment with his current attitude as it was a danger to patient care. When probed, the student eventually revealed that his father passed away in a similar ward environment and that he has been putting on a 'brave face' to just get through the placement; the student breaks down and cries. With the student's consent, this is shared with the practice supervisor and the practice assessor, and a plan is formed to support the student to meet their outcomes. The final summative meeting is quite a surprising event with the student almost a different person, so grateful for being challenged, the opportunity to improve, and become a better nurse. Tearful again. Staff were full of praise for change in attitude, his progression, and successfully achieving the outcomes to a good standard, eventually. Kamran displayed a complete change in attitude towards the learning process and resolving issues: a challenging but very rewarding process for all the staff involved. It is difficult to see a student so upset but sometimes you have to go backwards, to get to root of the problem, before you can move forwards.

 Things to Think About

- Personal matters are often at the root of a student's behaviour.
- What it's like to feel part of a team that have mutual respect even if you make an error.

 Applying Theory to Practice

- Building rapport helps the student to feel they can open up and express their feelings.

- Using the Thinking, Feeling, Acting model of coaching based on cognitive behaviour coaching can be a quick and simple intervention.
- Check the thinking errors list in Chapter 5 – we can all suffer from these and its crucial as a both supervisor and student to check in with yourself to see how you feel you are progressing.

 ## Exemplar of a Coaching Conversation

Signposting theory	Coaching conversation
Rapport building is essential to create the trust needed to encourage open and honest dialogue supported with open questioning.	**LL:** *Thanks for coming in to meet with me. I just felt we needed to clear the air and find out how you are feeling?*
Quickly opens to identify his feelings.	**Kamran:** *I'm still feeling upset.*
Using the cognitive behaviour model TFA (Chapter 5) to encourage Kamran to examine what thoughts are influencing his feelings and behaviour.	**LL:** *Tell me about what is going on in your head?*
Evidence of reflection indicting a possible thinking error of discounting positives and focusing on negatives.	**Kamran:** *I work hard, I study seriously, I take note of everything that is told to me but nothing I do is ever right?*
Using his language it is possible to get Kamran to expand further on what's going on for him in his head, heart, and action.	**LL:** *Nothing?*
Unhelpful thought and grief clearly communicated.	**Kamran:** *I try so hard and I have spent all this time studying instead of being with my family, in particular with my Dad who just died and for what? It looks like I will fail my qualification anyway!*
Empathy expressed genuinely and open question to extract what has been going on in Kamran's thinking.	**LL:** *It sounds as though you have had a really tough time. Tell me what's been going on for you Kamran?*
No challenge needed as you are collecting data to help Kamran help himself. Really important revelation that Kamran thinks that no one else believed in him other than his father.	**Kamran:** *It was only my father who believed in me, no one else really does.*

Signposting theory	Coaching conversation
Extracting the feeling but also highlighting the relationship between thoughts and feelings. People often mistake thoughts for facts and are unused to isolating them.	**LL:** *How does that make you feel thinking like that?*
Clearly unhelpful feelings.	**Kamran:** *Upset and angry.*
Follow through open questions on how feelings determine our actions.	**LL:** *And feeling upset and angry, how do you behave to your colleagues?*
Honest self-reflection identifying the possible impact on others and perceived rudeness that had been mentioned in the feedback.	**Kamran:** *With suspicion. Unfriendly even? Perhaps a bit provocative?*
Important to acknowledge the reflection in order to encourage other more helpful identification of feelings.	**LL:** *Well done with that honest look at yourself!* *Now have a think about how you want to feel?*
Kamran given the challenge easily identifies a more helpful positive thought.	**Kamran:** *Oh that's easy! Confident! In control.*
Further encouragement is the key to more helpful thinking needed to sustain the feelings and action.	**LL:** *Great! So what do you need to say to yourself that is going to help you feel confident and in control?*
Recognition that he is a work in progress similar to the rest of us! None of us are perfect; we all need help from time to time.	**Kamran:** *I am still learning and I have lots of support to get things right!*
Important to follow up with the consequences of thinking feeling and now identify what action he feels is needed in order to close the learning loop.	**LL:** *That sounds great Kamran; and what will you do as a result of thinking you are still learning and you have lots of support to get things right?*
Clear action identified.	**Kamran:** *Listen! Be observant. Learn more!*
In any coaching conversation if action is identified then a deadline needs to follow to ensure it happens.	**LL:** *When can you take this action?* **Kamran:** *Now!*
Tapping into the feelings is also helpful to motivate action.	**LL:** *How does that make you feel now?*
The evidence that coaching often brings something new: To think, to do, to feel.	**Kamran:** *Surprised that I can manage my thoughts to achieve a different feeling and actions!*

Self-Learning

Link Lecturer/Supervisor

- How confident would you feel about encouraging your students to be explicit about what is going on in their heads, hearts, and behaviour?
- What could you do to be even more confident to challenge your students in a positive productive style?
- How do you review what is going on in your head, heart, and behaviour as a supervisor?

Student

- It's easy to suffer from thinking errors (we all tend to) please check out Chapter 5 and ask yourself honestly, which do you feel you can identify with?
- If one of your colleagues were behaving in an unfriendly way, how would you support them?

Scenario 3: Solution-Focused Conversations and Supporting the Student's Emotional Intelligence to Help Turn a Negative Situation into Positive Learning

Anna feels quite confident about her progression on the placement and received good feedback at her formative assessment. She was encouraged to lead patient care under indirect supervision and take initiative where appropriate. With only two weeks left of the placement, things had been going very well until one shift. Anna was caring for Patient A who was admitted for substance misuse and disagreed with Sam's instructions not to share information with the patient. Patient A was on the ward for treatment but threatening to discharge himself. He had been moved to a side room and Sam had specifically told staff not to talk to him as he was being aggressive. Anna had disagreements with Sam on a number of previous occasions and generally found her difficult to talk to. However, on this occasion Anna felt Sam was being particularly harsh towards Patient A so asked to talk to the clinical educator when he came up to the ward. The clinical educator asked Sam for a meeting.

Things to Think About

- As the clinical educator, how would you carry out this conversation in a supportive way?
- Who supports the supervisors?
- How can Sam take away any learning from the situation?

Applying Theory to Practice

- Gestalt and NLP based coaching approaches embrace a holistic way of supporting learners whoever they are – students or supervisors. In this is example we will look at Perceptual Positioning or the Meta Mirror.
- As with most coaching interventions, we tend to use a sliver of theory, but there are always others we could have used.

Exemplar of a Coaching Conversation

Signposting theory	Coaching conversation
Setting the scene by being positive and honest.	**George:** *Thanks for joining me Sam – I have been told that you are having some difficulties with one of your students? And a patient?*
Sam is encouraged to identify the issue for herself and focuses on the student as the problem.	**Sam:** *Hi George, yes its Anna. She is an excellent student in many ways but has failed to follow my instructions on several occasions resulting in all sorts of difficulties and problems. The patient is another issue all together!*
Important to ask for permission but in a non-threatening way.	**George:** *OK Sam, just bear with me as I try something out with you?*
Agreement to participate helps gain buy-in to process.	**Sam:** *OK.*
Good open questioning extracting feelings.	**George:** *How does it make you feel when Anna disregards your instructions?*

Signposting theory	Coaching conversation
Feelings quickly identified.	**Sam:** *Annoyed and frustrated.*
The process of moving chairs is crucial as it helps change perspective within an individual.	**George:** *OK, thanks Sam; now if you could sit in this chair over here now? In this chair you are Anna – and so I want you to get into the heart and mindset of Anna.*
More evidence of participation.	**Sam:** *OK.*
Important to help the individual get into the mind and heart of the other person even if they don't know them that well.	**George:** *OK Anna, having listened to everything Sam has said today and previously how does that make you feel?*
Clear identification of feelings will help Sam gain further insight.	**Sam:** *Outraged! I am doing my best! A bit hurt really.*
This movement is crucial and for some people it takes them a while to think of a wise person so you can suggest they can use someone they have heard of or even their wisest self?	**George:** *OK, thanks Sam; now move to this third chair please. In this chair you are the wisest person you know.*
Very quick to think of her wisest person!	**Sam:** *Oh that would be my Mum!*
Important to talk and address the wise person with their name or title as this will help the individual locate their wise person within themselves.	**George:** *Good. OK Sam's Mum, having listened to Sam and to Anna, what have you learnt?*
Another outside perspective will help develop insight and understanding.	**Sam:** *Well that Sam is a bit fed up with Anna and Anna doesn't feel valued by Sam – in fact she feels outraged by the way Sam interacts with her.*
Important now for the wise person to give advice – this is really Sam giving herself advice with the lens of her Mum.	**George:** *OK, yes that sounds a fair assessment, and given your wisdom what advice would you give to Sam?*
Sounds like a good move forward.	**Sam:** *Sam you need to be more collaborative with Anna and demonstrate the benefits of working together in a team rather than against each other? Show her that you do rate her knowledge and skills?*

Signposting theory	Coaching conversation
Challenging the specifics here is crucial to get to the action. Even following coaching model GROW might be appropriate?	**George:** *OK Sam's Mum, and how would you suggest Sam did that?*
Sounds like this is a way of managing Thoughts, Feelings, and Actions approach.

Specific action to communicate how much Sam values Anna but needs to shape this dangerous tendency to break the rules. | **Sam:** *As my Mum knows me so well she would say believe in yourself Sam, you know what you are doing! You believe in Anna – tell her that, but also tell her that if she refuses to obey the procedures and protocols she will damage her potentially brilliant career!* |
Always good to check in with the feelings on the advice given and if time go round again as new data may emerge.	**George:** *Thanks Sam. Back in your chair now, what do you think about what your Mum is advising you now?*
Clear commitment communicated.	**Sam:** *Well she was a nurse too George, and I have shared loads with her, so I totally believe her advice to be sound.*
Always important to check with how your colleague is feeling to get insight into feelings for action needed.	**George***: OK Sam, how does that advice from your Mum make you feel now?*
Great result.	**Sam:** *Calm and together, thanks George. I feel a lot more confident about talking to Anna to achieve the result we need to. Thanks.*
Always good to end coaching conversations with asking this question.	**George:** *So, Sam, what are you taking away from this conversation?*
Reflective and focused to achieve a different outcome.

Involving Anna in finding a real way forward is more likely to last. | **Sam:** *A different perspective really. I was so focused on my own feelings of frustration I had lost sight of the influence I am still able to offer. I am going to talk to Anna now about boundaries, protocols, and benefits of procedures to her, and her patients, of following them. Asking her what she feels she needs to do to apply them.* |

Signposting theory	Coaching conversation
Always useful to review situations as things can change so quickly. Best to tackle one issue at a time rather than overwhelm colleagues with multiple issues.	**George:** *Great! Let's catch up in a couple of days to check in? Perhaps we can discuss progress with Patient A?*
Open and willing to review is further evidence that this conversation has been useful.	**Sam:** *Thanks, that would be really helpful.*

 ## Self-Learning

Supervisor
- What did you learn from this approach?
- What would you do differently?
- What needs to happen with following up on the conversation about Patient A?

Clinical Educator
- What did you learn from this approach?
- How could you apply this approach with colleagues?
- What do you need to develop for yourself to enable you to support the supervisors?

10

Community Nursing Case Study

Rachel Paul, Charlene Lobo and Theresa Walker

This case study is based on a 12-week placement with student nurses in the community. Although students are generally second year, there may be third year students on their final placements. It is expected that by the end of their placement the third-year students should be able to manage a full/almost full caseload and the second-year students will have an ability to assess, plan, implement, and evaluate basic level of care delivery independently, developing their autonomous practice.

The community trust in this case study divides its nursing workforce into teams that deliver planned care to clients within a contained postcode. Feeding into each team is the unplanned care team which in effect triages new cases and then passes on the care to the planned team, a community matron who will take referrals of patients with complex long-term conditions, and general practices within the identified post code area – all of which may also accommodate student placements. Students allocated to the community are generally buddied up and the pair allocated to one supervisor, which will be their main placement. The students are primarily allocated to the district nursing teams but are also placed with community matrons, the unplanned care team, general practice, and other specialist teams. Figure 10.1 demonstrates the community team for this case study on community nursing.

Usually there is a large number of students that go out to practice in the community, so a placement plan is set up for the whole period and the student overall experience is managed by the clinical educators. Students start their placement with a general induction day in the morning and

Collaborative Learning in Practice: Coaching to Support Student Learners in Healthcare, First Edition. Charlene Lobo, Rachel Paul, and Kenda Crozier.
© 2021 John Wiley & Sons Ltd. Published 2021 by John Wiley & Sons Ltd.
Companion website: www.wiley.com/go/lobo/collaborativelearninginpractice

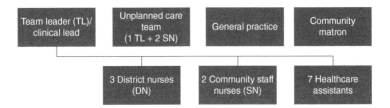

Figure 10.1 Community nursing team overview.

then go out to their practice areas and meet their supervisors. In the first couple of weeks, students will usually work one-to-one with their supervisors or other team members where they will spend the time acclimatising to community nursing, home visiting, and familiarising themselves with trust policies – especially in relation to home visiting and safeguarding. During this they will be assessed as to their learning needs, complete a first interview, and their supervisor should begin to put together a small caseload for the two students, roughly allocating four patients per student. The patients selected will usually require simple interventions such as simple dressings, skin care, catheter care, health promotion on managing chronic illnesses, etc. It is the supervisor's responsibility to gain consent from patients for students to deliver their care.

Community Nursing – City Team A

Figure 10.2 is a diagrammatic representation of City Team A that we are using in the community case study.

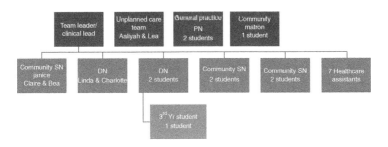

Figure 10.2 Community nursing team in detail.

Scenario 1: Unconfident Student, Overcoming Obstacles to Learning

Bea came to community placement with enthusiasm and confidence; however, over the course of the first two weeks, it became clear to Janice that she had become quiet and seemed disengaged when visiting patients with Janice. Bea's communication with patients was becoming increasingly limited. However, her buddy, Claire, seemed to be engaging with patients and their care.

Janice raised her concerns with Bea; Bea said that on the ward she felt confident and in her comfort zone. However, in patients' homes she was finding it hard as she felt she lost her skills and had to learn new ones, which made her feel less confident. She also felt very shocked in peoples' homes sometimes by the way they lived and the difficult situations they experienced.

 ## Things to Think About

- How would you conduct the conversation with Bea?
- How could you approach resolving this?
- How would you assess Bea? What criteria would you use? How would you evidence this?

 ## Applying Theory to Practice

This conversation is used as an example of how to raise a concern with a student. In this situation it is apparent that Bea's performance is not up to the expected standard for a second-year student. Janice is not sure what the issue is, but needs to act sooner rather than later and, taking a positive stance, her approach focuses on support as opposed to failure. When someone's performance is not as expected it's important to find the back-story to see what can be done. In Chapter 5 we looked at how cognitive behaviour coaching helps us to research the back-story – more importantly, it helps the student to research themselves. It's rare that people get a chance to look at their thoughts, feelings, and actions and helping them to do this will encourage your students to self-monitor and potentially manage themselves even more powerfully to achieve their goals. We often mistake thoughts for facts or feelings for facts so this model is an excellent start to help us to become more insightful in what we know and what we don't know.

 ## *Exemplar of a Coaching Conversation*

In a one-to-one with Bea, using a cognitive approach (thoughts, feelings, and actions) to coaching to try to uncover the issue.

Signposting the theory	Coaching dialogue
Keeping to an adult to adult relationship with an invitation to work together in collaboration.	**Janice:** *Thanks for joining me Bea and I wonder how you might feel us doing a bit of work together?*
Feels able to question back showing an equality in the relationship.	**Bea:** *What sort of work do you mean?*
Supervisor has clearly listened to the feelings as well as facts – an example of reflective listening.	**Janice:** *Some coaching work based on what you said to me earlier about how you were feeling now that you were working in patient's homes?*
A welcome clarification.	**Bea:** *What do you want me to do?*
Reminding the student that there are ground rules set to ensure confidential coaching and a safe environment to learn. This is particularly important when supporting students who learn differently, e.g. with dyslexia. Bea doesn't; but what would you do for a student if they did?	**Janice:** *Just to work with me please Bea. Remember when we work together what you say to me is confidential, there are no right or wrongs, I'm just here to focus on supporting your learning.*
	Bea: *OK. Where do we start?*
The reason Janice has chosen to use TFA (cognitive coaching approach) is because of the feelings divulged. Feelings are often a result of unhelpful thoughts and can lead to unhelpful actions, so it's good to nip them in the bud.	**Janice:** *I have a piece of paper and pen here. Divide the page into these three headings: Thoughts, Feelings, Actions. This is all about researching yourself.*

Signposting the theory	Coaching dialogue
Bea is clearly open and reflective thanks to the safe environment created by Janice and by engaging is taking ownership of researching herself with some encouragement from Janice in the form of listening, questioning, and feedback.	**Bea:** *OK – here we go.*
By being able to express her depth of feeling and the variety of unhelpful thoughts, the real difficulties Bea is experiencing are made more transparent. Quite often people feel embarrassed to reveal their thoughts and feelings like this and it is down to the rapport built by the supervisor as to how effective this is. Bea is currently unable to take action.	**Janice:** *Under the feelings heading just note down how you are feeling working in a patient's house? Perhaps use your most uncomfortable experience?* Bea quickly notes down embarrassed, and then adds uncomfortable.
Again, returning to the feelings aspects of TFA, Janice can work more deeply to support Bea in managing her feelings, thoughts, and actions. Coaching tools like TFA are to be made transparent so the students can not only understand what the supervisor is doing but they can use the tools for themselves on their own. Great self-awareness! Silence is good! The more silence the more time the students have to reflect and make sense of their learning.	**Janice:** *OK Bea, well done, now remember these notes belong to you and you take them away – what is the thought that went on in your head when you felt embarrassed or uncomfortable? Please note that down on the paper?* Bea notes down – It's really dirty in this house! – this patient lives, sleeps, and eats in the chair! How does anyone live like this? It's so dirty, I don't want to touch anything, I don't know where to put down my equipment, I don't know where to sit or how to manage a dressing in such dirty conditions.

Signposting the theory	Coaching dialogue
Genuine acknowledgement develops rapport.	**Janice:** *Thanks Bea. When you were feeling these things and thinking these things, what did you do as a result?* Bea notes down – 'nothing' and 'I clam up'; under actions, 'Charlotte took over'. **Janice:** *How did you feel about that Bea?* Bea added 'useless – community not my thing' to the feelings column.
Supervisor used the list of thinking errors.	**Janice: (shows Bea a list of thinking errors)** *OK Bea; so we all have what are known as thinking errors, thoughts that are unsubstantiated by fact which influence our thinking and actions in a negative way. When you look at this list of thinking errors, ones that we all have from time to time, perhaps you can identify one behind your conclusion that 'community is not your thing?'*
Bea reassured that everyone has thinking errors is more comfortable to identify hers. Supervisor is transparent about the process in order to encourage Bea to use it on herself.	**Bea:** *Ah these ones! OK, discounting the positives?* **Janice:** *OK – as you can see our thoughts feelings and actions are all linked together. What we don't always do is write them out quite like this, but it can really help to explain what is going on.* **Bea:** *I hadn't realised that.*

Signposting the theory	Coaching dialogue
By acknowledging that the thought is based on an unhelpful assumption, Janice can explore what Bea enjoys about working in the community?	**Janice:** *How does it help you acknowledging you might be discounting the positives of community?*
Great insight as a result of the coaching.	**Bea:** *That I have been letting these feelings and thoughts get on top of me! Not caring for my patients.*
Encourage positive reflection.	**Janice:** *What do you enjoy about working in the community?*
Reflecting on the positives of community is a potential source of motivation for Bea.	**Bea:** *The informality – building relationships that make such a difference to often long-term patients.*
Summarise and evaluate.	**Janice:** *OK Bea, so that sounds like you have gained some good insight. We all have a choice in what we think, feel, and how we act. What might be a more helpful thought in this situation?* There is a long pause. Silence is good, it is always too tempting to fill in the space!
Bea identified a more helpful thought.	**Bea:** *Perhaps if I say to myself* **think about the patient.**
	Janice: (Nods and smiles) *Yes of course; if you are saying to yourself think about the patient, how will that make you feel?*
	Bea: (Looks thoughtful) *It will help me focus on care and be a bit more positive and optimistic!*

Signposting the theory	Coaching dialogue
Making clear we do all have a choice in how we think, feel and act is potentially empowering!	**Janice:** *OK Bea; so feeling a bit more positive and optimistic, what action might you take?*
	Bea: (Looks less anxious) *I will look at each patient and find something positive and nice to say about them.*
	Janice: *Brilliant – and how will that make you feel?*
Always set a date!	**Bea:** *Better, more positive, not dreading visiting patients at home*
	Janice: *And when will you start this?*
	Bea: *Tomorrow!*

Self-Learning

Compare this conversation to the notes you made in the 'think about' section. What are the similarities and the differences? Note how the positive supportive mindset/perspective influences the language and tone of the conversation.

Go to the companion website to see an example of Bea's assessment.

How the Situation Was Resolved

Using the community-led Leg Ulcer Clinic (LUC), where patients come to clinic for their treatment in conjunction with home visits; first Bea met and assisted with several patients who attended the LUC during the week (in a hospital/clinical setting) and then at the weekend visited the same patients at home for their dressing change, initially accompanying the registered nurse. This plan helped Bea to build a relationship with the patient in a clinical setting before meeting them in their home, giving her more time and experience to build confidence and overcome her anxiety about nursing in a community setting.

Scenario 2: Team Discord, Facilitating Teamworking

It is week 6 of this community placement and Mary has noticed that on joint visits to patients Aaliyah often leads on the visit with limited input from Lea; sometimes it is clear that Aaliyah has taken over the lead for Lea's caseload. When working one-to-one with Lea, Mary has found that Lea is very quiet and reticent in care delivery, a view that is supported by feedback from some of the other supervisors.

 Things to Think About

- What might the issues be?
- What are the implications of doing nothing?
- How would you explore different perspectives?

 Applying Theory to Practice

We need to do something here in the first instance to investigate what is going on. Aaliyah's view might be that she finds Lea lacks motivation, there is a personality clash, lacks appropriate knowledge. Lea might feel overpowered by Aaliyah's enthusiasm, feels bullied, has different learning needs/styles. As a coach we might need to find out what are the two perspectives here and we need to explore perceptual positioning.

Perceptual positioning is a great tool from the NLP (Neuro Linguistic Programming) stable of tools, as discussed in Chapter 5. This challenge of moving chairs is easier if you as the supervisor trust and believe in the process. You are more likely to see the benefits for the student and yourself after you have completed using perceptual positioning!

The intention of individual sessions with both Aaliyah and Lea is to help each student gain greater perspective on how each of them may be affecting the other and to take action to overcome the difficulties they are perceived as having. It is a useful tool to use when coaching for teamworking as it builds on developing respectfulness and valuing each other. In the example below we considered conducting this conversation individually to start with, in order to explore different perspectives with the use of perceptual positioning and build a more effective working relationship between Aaliyah and Lea.

 ## *Exemplar of a Coaching Conversation*

Signposting the theory	Coaching dialogue
Gentle persuasion to try something new? Reminder of all important ground rules.	**Mary:** *Just bear with me Aaliyah I want to try something out with you? Bear in mind we are working with the same ground rules we normally do.*
Good for student to recall the ground rules rather than just be told them by the supervisor	**Aaliyah:** *OK, yes I know! Confidentiality, honesty, and openness.*
Focus first on extracting the feeling Feeling reveals what Aaliyah is thinking too.	**Mary:** *How does working with Lea make you feel?*
Negativity clearly revealed – when assumptions are voiced they are more easily challenged.	**Aaliyah:** *Annoyed! Lea is always trying to get out of doing anything and just leaves me to do it all!*
Supervisor has to persist in extracting the feelings.	**Mary:** *And how does that make you feel?*
This is quite a challenge – the difficulty is made worse if the individual has no empathy for the other person.	**Aaliyah:** *Well I don't care now – it's her look out as I'm the one progressing well and getting my work signed off and Lea is getting nowhere!*
Sometimes it takes a couple of goes round the cycle for people to see a different perspective?	**Mary:** *OK, thanks; now go and sit in that chair over there?* *In that chair you are Lea. Just get into your head and heart what you know about her.*

Signposting the theory	Coaching dialogue
Getting Aaliyah to see things from Lea's perspective is crucial as is looking at the feelings identified.	**Mary:** *OK Lea, you have listened to everything Aaliyah has said – not just today but previously too – how does that make you feel?*
OK, so Aaliyah is beginning to acknowledge that Lea doesn't have as much confidence when talking to patients.	**Aaliyah** (as Lea): *A bit upset really, we used to be good friends, but Aaliyah is so much more confident than me and I feel so nervous when talking to patients.*
Focusing on a completely different perspective to learn from.	**Mary:** *OK, thanks; please sit in that third chair now?*
Learner reflects positive rapport with supervisor using gentle humour.	**Aaliyah:** *This is a good workout for me!*
This is a crucial perspective and encourages the learner to see the situation from a different perspective generating even greater learning.	**Mary:** *Absolutely!* *Now in this third chair think of the wisest person you know or have heard of?*
Personal choice of the wise person will give greater impact to learning identified as well as advice. Of course in reality this is just Aaliyah – but her 'wisest' or 'best' self.	**Aaliyah:** *Ok that's easy! My Gran!* **Mary:** *OK Aaliyah's Gran, what have you learned from listening to these two?*
Connection to possible feelings is the breakthrough in developing greater empathy for Lea.	**Aaliyah** (as Gran): *OK, well they are both feeling a bit upset really! Lea feels sad she has lost a friend and a bit left behind by Aaliyah.*
Advice giving from within! Essentially Aaliyah is telling herself what to do.	**Mary:** *OK, and so as the wise person, what would you advise Aaliyah to do?*
Aaliyah has identified what she feels might help her friend and because she is making use of everything that she knows about her friend it is more likely to work.	**Aaliyah:** *Ok that is a bit harder…* *I know! Aaliyah can ask Lea what she wants her to do, to help her? Perhaps even remind her that she is brilliant with things like detail – and how they make a good team, as Aaliyah can't always remember the detail like her?*
Keep instructions focused and simple.	**Mary:** *OK, Aaliyah; perhaps move back now into your first chair where you were you?*

Signposting the theory	Coaching dialogue
Go with the rapport building.	**Aaliyah:** *This reminds me of musical chairs!*
Need to confirm and remind the learner what it is they agreed to do and how.	**Mary:** *So back in your original chair, how does what the wise person has said and advised you to do make you feel?*
The connection is developed and empathy clearly apparent resulting in compassionate support and action.	**Aaliyah:** *OK – actually it reminds me that although we are very different, we used to get on really well. As I did more, so Lea withdrew and has become really quiet. Perhaps if I find out from Lea what I can do to help her do more she will grow more in confidence? Then we might both feel happier working together? It might be slightly tricky having that conversation with Lea!*
Acknowledgement of feelings but a chance to review what has helped in previous tricky conversations.	**Mary:** *Possibly. When you have had slightly tricky conversations previously, what has helped you?*
Action identified based on previous experience of what worked previously.	**Aaliyah:** *Planning what I will say and practising them with a friend!*
Always good to look at when the action will happen.	**Mary:** *So, when could your conversation take place?*
Specific time and place identified making the action more likely to be a reality.	**Aaliyah:** *After our shift today?*
Follow through on this is crucial to ensure action is taken.	**Mary:** *Great; and how will you feel having this conversation?*
The benefits of the action are clearly articulated making it more likely to be taken.	**Aaliyah:** *This is a real chance to build back my friendship with Lea and keep reminding myself that as my Gran says, sometimes I can get carried away and forget the impact I have on other people?*
Always a checking in opportunity.	**Mary:** *Great! Let me know how you get on?*

Self-Learning

- How do you feel about facilitating the use of perceptual positioning?
- Where could you go to for support in developing your skills and confidence in using this approach?
- What would you value about using this approach?
- Have a go and try to formulate a conversation between the supervisor and Lea.
- As a clinical educator: how would you support a supervisor who came to you for support? What would you need to do to better develop your skills to support supervisors?
- As an assessor: how would the feedback influence your judgement on the student's assessment?

Go to the companion website to see Aliyah and Lea's learning logs.

Scenario 3: Using Coaching Approaches in a Crisis

Linda and Charlotte are in their 8th week of placement and have got their caseload. They visited Mrs F for a planned leg wound dressing, they had seen her before with their supervisor Rob for the initial assessment and treatment planning. Both students and supervisor were confident they had the skill level and competency to continue visiting on their own.

On visiting Mrs F, both students quickly realised she was in an acute critical condition, as she was pale and clammy, very short of breath, but conscious and could barely speak. They took her observations and rang 999. Whilst waiting for the ambulance, Linda reassured and comforted Mrs F and Charlotte phoned Rob, who came immediately as he was close by.

Mrs F was admitted to the acute hospital, Linda and Charlotte secured the house with Rob, and Rob informed relatives of events.

Things to Think About

- As a supervisor, if this happened to you, what would you feel?
- How would you conduct the telephone conversation in order to decide your actions? What are the issues you think you would be considering?
- As the supervisor, how would you de-brief Linda and Charlotte when they return to the health centre?

Applying Theory to Practice

In this scenario, we are looking at supervising students in a very highly emotionally charged situation. There are three important issues that we are looking at here.

Firstly, how do we conduct this conversation? This incident where emotions are highly charged is a good reminder to us as both supervisors and learners that our ability to listen and keep calm depends on our personal mindset. Various theories (emotional intelligence/drama and winners triangle/transactional analysis/cognitive behaviour coaching) are all good reminders – discussed in Chapter 5 –that help reinforce the relationship between our core skills of coaching and our state of mind.

A second important aspect of this case is to consider de-briefing the students when they return to base. The aims of the de-briefing are to clarify what learning both Linda and Charlotte can take away from this visit to Mrs F. The incident held crucial learning for all involved. As learning takes place in real life or death situations it is essential to unpick the learning from incidents to ensure that all steps and protocols were strictly followed and clear reasoning for actions offered to embed learning. By focusing on the outcomes needed for the patient, Mrs F, and any actions taken or not taken, the learning can potentially be made even more powerful. A question that springs to mind here is: what learning can you take away from this incident?

The third significant issue to consider here is how we support students to develop resilience through adverse situations. However, this will be covered in-depth in another scenario.

There could be two very different endings: which one do you feel would be effective in supporting learning?

 ## *Exemplar of Response 1 – Command and Control*

Rob turns up immediately and takes control of the situation. Linda and Charlotte are so relieved to see Rob and immediately hand responsibility over to him. They follow his orders and after the incident feel both grateful and appreciative of Rob stepping in and sorting everything out for them. On reflection, they felt they could have just left Rob to it. They perceived there wasn't anything they could do, so they felt slightly redundant, reinforcing existing self-doubt and reducing confidence.

In this response it seemed like Rob was saying to himself:

> *These students are too inexperienced to cope with this situation: this is a medical emergency and I need to take over as I don't trust them to know what to do!*

As a result, Linda and Charlotte quickly picked up on that feeling, with lack of confidence resulting in a mirroring of low levels of confidence in their capabilities. *'If Rob doesn't trust me then I don't trust myself!'* Belief in the students to know what they needed to do would have encouraged them to take the much needed action. The questioning that Rob undertook in the telephone conversation did not convince or reassure him that Linda and Charlotte knew what to do.

It is only natural that as supervisors we want to be seen as the source of much valued knowledge, and we may also be used to being in a rescue mode. This does not necessarily encourage learners to think for themselves or step up to take responsibility or accountability for learning from decisions made. When we ask closed or leading questions, we limit the range of information we get to make adequate assessments. In learning situations such as the one outlined, it may have been really hard for Rob not to give feedback to Linda and Charlotte. They were feeling stressed and desperate for support so the natural instinct of Rob was to give that support and tell them what to do.

Exemplar of Response 2 – Coaching

On the phone, Rob used open coaching questions to ascertain whether this was an incident that they had experienced before, what they had already done, and what they were planning to do next. Rob carefully noted that both Linda and Charlotte had previous relevant experience, had acted according to all protocols and were completely confident that they knew what to do next. Rob gave them specific positive feedback on what they had achieved and asked them both how they were feeling. After being told that – although initially they had felt concerned after carrying out the actions and protocols – they now felt in control of the situation, Rob reflected back on what they told him, including their feelings about their next steps, and actions were agreed and taken.

In the case of response 2, Rob may have reflected not just on previous experience and relevant situations that Linda and Charlotte had experienced, but also how they felt about their skills to deal with the current situation. Reflective listening is where you demonstrate you have really taken in all the information including the feelings presented. Reflective listening is as crucial as questioning in coaching, if not more so, in my experience.

This summary will have also served an additional purpose of giving Linda and Charlotte the opportunity to listen to themselves again, another opportunity to check that they really did feel they knew what to do and were in control of the situation. This builds the intrinsic motivation of learners – as they begin to trust themselves based on the questioning and reflective listening skills of their coach or supervisor.

Self-Learning

- With response 1, how much learning would Linda and Charlotte be able to identify?
- With response 2, what was the impact of the coaching approach?
- Have a go at framing a coaching conversation that Rob would use with the students on the telephone in response 2.

What Made This Incident Important to Learn From?

Preferring to be self-directing and in control over their learning, the de-briefing offers a collaborative opportunity to support Linda and Charlotte to review honestly and openly without judgement their individual roles, within the incident, encouraging them to reflect and solve real-life problems and grow their confidence and capabilities as developing professionals. The de-brief makes the learning meaningful as most adults are interested in real-life learning and motivated to be even better when faced with a similar issue as part of their desire to grow and progress.

Compare response 1 and 2 in how the incident was used to develop learning.

Clear Acknowledgement of Their Own Life Experiences as a Basis for Learning

Starting off with the question "When has something similar happened to you before?" gave Rob the opportunity to find out that Linda and Charlotte had experienced something similar before, which meant they were able to discuss past actions and knowledge of relevant protocols. The de-brief gives both learners the opportunity to reflect further on their life and work experiences so far, surfacing potentially relevant facts and feelings before binding them together with new learning.

Using the de-brief to highlight key learning to resolve a real-life problem, in this case the response to Mrs F and a possible cardiac arrest, Linda and Charlotte have applied past learning and under response 2 confidently carried out their actions, reinforcing good practice – with the support of Rob who after careful questioning was able to trust and believe in his two able students to use their learning. In response 1, Rob did not use his questioning and listening to uncover the existing knowledge and experience, thereby limiting both the learning and confidence building needed to grow his students.

Learners are potentially motivated by a sense of purpose and an intrinsic desire to develop themselves; as supervisors and trainers, it is up to us to encourage this intrinsic motivation.

What are the ways that you encourage the intrinsic motivation of your students?

 Go to the companion website to see Linda's learning log.

11

Maternity Case Study

Kenda Crozier, Rachel Paul and Charlene Lobo

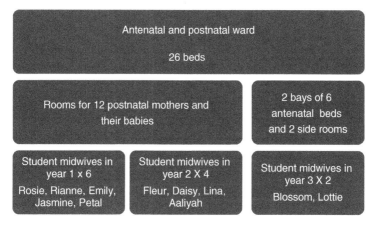

The ward has one midwife coordinating and two to three midwives per shift to care for the women on the ward. There are four maternity support workers who provide delegated care and also support for breastfeeding.

There is a clinical educator called Maeve, who works Monday to Friday covering this ward, the delivery suite, and the midwifery-led unit. The clinical educator has worked with the ward to plan the student rota and has supported the staff to develop collaborative ways of working. The NMC (2018.1.5) standards for student supervision and assessment expect that 'there is a nominated person for each practice setting to actively support students and address student concerns'. In this setting, Maeve as clinical educator takes on this role.

The duty rota for the first week has been supplied by the university placements team along with a link to the student welcome pack.

Rosie is a first-year student who has been on the programme for six months. She is in module 2 of her first year and theory has focused on labour and normal physiological birth, antenatal care, and basic skills in clinical observations to assess well-being in women and newborn infants. In the first module, she was placed on the delivery suite for four weeks, then in community for four weeks. She is now beginning a five-week placement and is nervous because she is unsure of her clinical skills.

Fleur is a second-year student who has undertaken her first-year placements in another hospital trust and is in the second half of her second year. The first placement of year 2 was spent on community and in the midwife-led birthing unit. Fleur is not familiar with the ward and is still getting used to the paper recordkeeping because her previous trust used electronic records for everything.

Blossom is third-year student who is looking forward to qualifying in six months' time. She has been on the ward for two weeks before the first- and second-year students arrive, so is familiar with the routine and the staff. She is comfortable in her abilities and feels confident.

She has been a peer supporter for breastfeeding and draws on that knowledge. She is active in a few local and online discussion forums for mums and has a tendency to draw on knowledge from conversations in those groups to give advice to women.

Rosie, Fleur, and Blossom have been in placement together in the first part of this academic year. NMC SSSA (2018) states that students should be empowered to be proactive and take responsibility for their learning (statement 1.7) and that learning should be tailored to the student stage of learning, focusing on outcome (statement 1.10).

Scenario 1: Balancing Student-Led Learning and Client Care Needs

On day one, Rosie arrives on time for her day shift; Fleur, Rosie, and Blossom are all allocated to the same bay in the antenatal ward under the supervision of Jenny. When they arrive, all staff are at the station and handover begins. Rosie is a bit lost with the speed of information but hopes she will be able to fill in the gaps later.

After handover Jenny, who is their supervisor today, greets Rosie and Fleur and tells them they are allocated to one antenatal care bay which is their learning environment. The bay contains six women who are all in the third trimester of pregnancy. Blossom is already in the bay greeting the women.

Jenny: *Nice to meet you both. My name is Jenny and I'm a staff midwife. I am going to be supervising you both and Blossom today in this antenatal bay ... not sure how that is going to go but please come and find me and ask me any questions if you need to, or check with Blossom as she has been here for a while and knows how things work. How did you find the handover? Did you understand everything?*

So, Fleur *I think you can go ahead and do the observations for Aesha Jones. Remember that she has pre-eclampsia so what are the important things to keep an eye on?*

Fleur: *Blood pressure and urinalysis?*

Jenny: *What else?*

Fleur: *Ummm ...*

Jenny: *Blurred vision or visual disturbances, headache. OK, look up the guidelines and the notes, make sure you check everything. Rosie, you can come with me and we will make a start.*

 ## Things to Think About

- What sort of information do students need when they are new to an area and how do you manage the introduction to learning opportunities?
- How might you, as the supervisor, broach the situation with students who are at different stages in their professional learning? This could be an actual experience or a hypothetical proposal on how you might manage such a situation.
- How can the students work together to support each other's learning, ensuring they meet their own learning outcomes?

 ## Applying Theory to Practice

The conversation in the scenario reflects a very task-focused perspective and could adopt a coaching approach based on the principles of coaching, namely the fourth principle – the student sets the agenda (see Chapter 5). At a first meeting at the beginning of the shift it is important to establish rapport, be explicit about expectations/boundaries/ground rules, and identify what learning outcomes are to be achieved. There is an opportunity to help students learn about working collaboratively. Everyone learns differently and the supervisor needs to know how they can facilitate learning for everyone. In keeping with the CLiP model it is good practice to set up a timeline for the day so it is agreed at which points students should check in with each other and with the supervisor.

Below is an exemplar of how a coaching conversation might be conducted in this scenario.

 ## Exemplar of a Coaching Conversation

Signposting the theory	Coaching dialogue
Beginning of the shift:	
Open question probing for feelings to start with so that learners can openly feedback.	**Jenny:** *Hi, how are you both feeling after the handover?*
Evidence of rapport as Rosie is open about her feelings.	**Rosie:** *A bit lost as everyone seems to know what they are doing here except me!*
Learner is also able to express her difficulties.	**Fleur:** *This is so different from how I have done things before!*
Empathic response communicating safety – essential for any learning – link to Maslow's intrinsic needs of motivation.	**Blossom:** *I remember feeling like that Rosie, but as soon as you get going you will be fine too.*
Start of a collaborative team meeting.	
Facilitates discussion on desired Outcome or Goal – using OSCAR or GROW templates from Chapter 5.	**Jenny:** *What outcome or goal would each of you like to achieve from the shift today?*
Lots of adult learners feel self-doubt, reassurance from peers as well as supervisors will make a real difference to building confidence.	**Rosie:** *I really don't know where to start. I need to practise how to do observations. Can I just watch you Jenny?*

Signposting the theory	Coaching dialogue
Felt encouraged to share positive action to settle into a new ward. Rosie as a first year can buddy up with Fleur which will hopefully increase confidence in questioning, listening, and new learning.	**Fleur:** *Come with me Rosie, let's take a look round the ward and find out where everything is so that if we need to get something we won't have to keep asking. The layout of the ward looks similar to the hospital I was in last year but things might be in a different place so it would be good to do it together. Then we are in a good position to learn the routines, protocols, and guidelines used on this ward.*
	Jenny: *OK, sounds like a good start. I don't know where Blossom has got to but we'll catch up again mid-morning.*

Checking in later in the shift:

Good open question.	**Jenny:** *How are you all getting on?*
Reflective listening evidence of some key learning, learning it's OK to feel a bit nervous clearly helped Rosie feel more at ease in revealing her feelings.	**Rosie:** *It's OK, I'm not so nervous. I've been working with Fleur doing observations and have got a better sense of what I am doing. I was finding out from the women and their records about their pregnancies and complications.*
Checking on progress towards the goals set for the shift. Open questioning to check learning.	**Jenny:** *What learning outcomes are you hoping to achieve from this first shift Fleur?*
The familiarity with new ways of doing things in a new hospital environment has started leaving room for new learning opportunities for Fleur.	**Fleur:** *I started to make new connections and feel more familiar with the systems and protocols I need to follow in this hospital ward. As Rosie said, we are working together.*
Open question used to encourage Fleur to take stock of her learning and in doing so repeat or embed learning and good practice from the day.	**Jenny:** *What have you learned about antenatal care delivery with the women in your care today?*
Fleur reflects on her learning and action.	**Fleur:** *The women I have met today seem to be excited and nervous about becoming new Mums. I was surprised they didn't know each other so I tried my best to encourage them to chat to each other and build connections.*

Signposting the theory	Coaching dialogue
Double question here, which could have backfired but luckily didn't as Blossom being confident gave an answer to both questions.	**Jenny:** *What about you Blossom, remind me what was it you needed to achieve in this shift?*
Whilst Blossom reflected carefully about her practice during the day and dealing with a mum that wasn't under her care, what is missing was the focus on what Blossom was supposed to be concentrating on, which was antenatal care.	**Blossom:** *I wanted to ensure that I could give breastfeeding support. I am writing my dissertation on motivating women to breastfeed so wanted to see if what I have been reading can be applied to practice. So I went over to the postnatal rooms and found a mum to talk to. I know she was not 'my woman' but Lottie didn't mind and the poor mum was just in tears and feeling like she couldn't do it. So I spent a good hour with her and just talked her through it. She needed to be kind to herself and we worked out the best position for her to be in to feed and the baby latched on. We just sat there and talked it through.*
Blossom is trying to wriggle out of facing up to the fact that she has deviated from the outcomes agreed.	*I've written up some evidence for you to sign about my achievements of learning outcomes Jenny.*
Adult-to-adult challenge – neutral non-judgemental approach that is genuinely curious to problem solve with Blossom a solution-focused approach to taking responsibility for her antenatal responsibilities and outcomes.	**Jenny:** *Blossom, let's spend some time together working out a way of achieving the outcome you had identified as being a priority? Let's talk after this meeting?*
Adult response.	**Blossom:** *OK, I get that – thanks.*
Notice the positive language in Jenny's question.	**Jenny:** *OK. Let me recap what I have heard. Rosie and Fleur you have been acclimatising yourselves to the ward and routine which is a really good starting point to do together. What other goals do you want to achieve by the end of the shift? Blossom, let's spend time now to discuss your evidence and review the plan on antenatal care to meet those outcomes.*
Engaging the team in taking responsibility for what they want to achieve and identifying what they need to do that.	
It is as important to look at what went well and what could be even better moving forward from one shift to the next.	

Self-Learning

Supervisor

- Having read this conversation, what is your learning and what action could you take as a result to become an even more empowering supervisor?
- How might you challenge a student to encourage focus on the care of the women she has been allocated, while considering balancing care needs and learning needs?

Remember that as a practice supervisor you are expected to contribute to the student's record of achievement, it is therefore important to have some clarity about the learning outcomes to be achieved for each shift. The way this is done may vary but there should be sufficient evidence to demonstrate to the practice assessor the extent to which the learner is meeting the outcomes of the programme according to the stage of their programme. You should be able to have opportunities to share your observations with the practice assessor.

Student

- What are the steps you take to familiarise yourself when starting on a new ward and a new module?
- What goals do you set and how do you ensure these are achieved?
- When and how are 'ground rules' communicated and agreed?
- What is your responsibility as a student in achieving success with your studies?

Timeline for the Student Journey

Each programme is slightly different and the learning journey is different for all individuals. Sometimes there may be learners from more than one university or education institution and from different programmes. As a supervisor or assessor you should consider how to encourage students to share where they are on their professional journey. They should be able to supply detail on what they have done on previous placements and show you evidence of their learning development and areas they need to work on further.

Scenario 2: Increasing Confidence

Blossom is now in the fifth week of this allocation, for Fleur and Rosie it is the end of their third week. The clinical educator Maeve arrives on the ward at 10.00. The students have been working together in one antenatal bay. She gathers all the students together and asks the midwife in charge if she can take them to work with her for an hour. She begins with an exercise to establish some ground rules.

During this learning hour they review the care they have provided and she offers them the chance to ask questions. Just before they return to the ward, Rosie asks to speak on her own to Maeve; Rosie brings out a list of terms and abbreviations that she has not understood. She asks Maeve to give her definitions of the terms.

Things to Think About

- How can Rosie be supported?
- How would you manage this situation using a coaching approach?
- How as a clinical educator might you support these students to learn together?

Applying Theory to Practice

This is an opportunity to consider how, as a supervisor, you would assess Rosie's learning needs.

Solutions-focused conversations focus on an individual's skills, strengths, and qualities that they can use to achieve the outcome they determine or see as needed. The initial meeting between supervisor and student provides an excellent opportunity for the supervisor to pick up information on that individual. How best to work with them, what metaphors may work with them, their strengths, qualities, and the values that they reveal. The initial meeting is sometimes called a 'chemistry' meeting or problem free chat where you get to know the individual first. The 'chemistry' may or may not be a luxury that can be afforded. We also believe that it's up to the supervisor to park his or her feelings as far as possible, as the relationship in coaching needs to be egalitarian. This might pose a challenge in a hierarchical culture. Parking our emotions as a supervisor is crucial to support the practice of reflective listening and the use of clean language, described in Chapter 5, which is where we avoid trying to influencing or leading the student.

 ## Exemplar of a Coaching Conversation Using Solutions-Focused Approach: OSCAR

Signposting the theory	Coaching dialogue
Open question to help Rosie identify what she needs from this tutorial time.	**Maeve:** *What do you want to achieve in this time?*
Outcome identified.	**Rosie:** *I have a whole list of terms and abbreviations that I haven't understood, please can you tell me what they all mean?*
Situation.	**Maeve:** *Well, yes, I could Rosie, but you have already been told them all at some point, what they all mean, and actually if you found them out for yourself how might that help you?*
Almost a childlike demand.	**Rosie:** *Well it would be quicker and less trouble if you just told me!*
Collaborating rather than becoming a parent helping Rosie look for other **choices.**	**Maeve:** *Quick learning doesn't always stick! What helps you to learn?*
Evaluation the **consequences** of those choices.	**Rosie:** *Well I like learning from doing things and making my own way of remembering things. Actually, I have designed all sorts of methods to remember procedures so far using a clock face!*
Helping Rosie expand and develop the **choices** she makes.	**Maeve:** *That sounds brilliant Rosie; so you've worked out how to remember once you have learned them, what other options do you have here to learn these terms and abbreviations?*

Signposting the theory	Coaching dialogue
Action identified by Rosie.	**Rosie:** *Well I could ask some of the other students?*
Encouraging Rosie to think of the implications.	**Maeve:** *What might the consequence of that be?*
Assess the situation realistically.	**Rosie:** *Everybody is very busy, and they don't ever seem to stop long enough for me to ask them anything.*
Persistence and patience – belief that Rosie will find the answers for herself.	**Maeve:** *Yes, they are busy, but where else could you find this information?*
It may seem an obvious solution, but the point is that Rosie identified it, so that it reflects her commitment to make it happen and own the action. More of an adult-to-adult conversation leading to collaboration.	**Rosie:** *I could look at my portfolio at the class notes about antenatal conditions like pre-eclampsia and in the trust guidelines, I guess. I make mind maps with different colours. In the last placement I made flash cards to remind me what various acronyms meant. I kept those in my portfolio and I looked at them all the time until I could remember the ones we used most often.*
Example of summative listening and open solutions-focused question	**Maeve:** *It sounds to me as though you have some good experience to draw on that helped you learn previously. How can that help you here?*
Good reflection.	**Rosie:** *I like to understand what I need to do and when. I am not good with written lists but find visual prompts like a sort of timeline reassuring and calming. That helps me think about what I need to do and when on a shift otherwise I get flustered.*
Open question to extract more information. Good observation from Maeve to pick up on Rosie's nervousness.	**Maeve:** *What else helps you to overcome any nervousness?*
Further reflection on what she feels she needs.	**Rosie:** *Having a private quiet place to think!*
Positive encouragement to identify a similar environment.	**Maeve:** *OK, good, where have you found this in the past?*

Signposting the theory	Coaching dialogue
Rosie knows where to take herself to calm herself and think.	**Rosie:** *An empty room on the ward or sometimes I have gone to the chapel on my way back from the canteen. The coffee room is too noisy with other people there.*
Evidence of active listening and positive feedback. Leaving the door open for support if and when needed.	**Maeve:** *Sounds like you have a great plan! Well done! What do you need from me?*
Positive outcome and feels comfortable to get support as and when needed. An opportunity to **review** the action and outcome.	**Rosie:** *Thanks! I'm not sure but I will let you know how I get on at our next tutorial.*

 ## *Self-Learning*

This offers an opportunity for you as a **supervisor** to reflect your current practice position and what you currently do to support students who may be on the autism spectrum.

People on the autistic spectrum find group sessions incredibly difficult and it would be unlikely that this client would gain any benefit. It really sounds as through Rosie could benefit from some specific one-to-one help. Her reactions should then be different. For her to develop other responses, it might help to work with her to define her strengths or list what she knows. This will probably be quite factual if she is on the spectrum, as 'they' don't see the softer skills as important. She could then be developed on the best ways to pass those skills on. The language will have to stay very 'clean' or the client won't 'get it'. Another angle may be to ask what she wants to be good at and then look at the current gap. Developing a plan to close the gap could follow this. I have made flash cards for some of my students to remind them of what to say in certain situations. Another student developed a visual flowchart for herself around conversations.

Some students on the spectrum react badly in a stress situation. Rosie may have been fearful that she was out of her comfort zone, so working out an escape route where she can sit safely and comfortably by herself might be an option to consider. A coaching conversation with Maeve needs to help Rosie feel safe to articulate her needs, fears, and strategies for supporting her overcoming them.

As a **student,** given a lot of us are on this spectrum, have a think about how best you learn.

There are free online questionnaires, but essentially there are four styles of learning based on the work of Dewey, Lewin, and Kolb, which are set out in Wildflower and Brennan (2011: p. 76):

1. The Activist: these are people who learn best from doing things – direct experience.
2. The Reflector: these are people who need some time to think about the impact of action.
3. The Theorist: who feels most comfortable with examining theory or principles underpinning any action.
4. The Pragmatist: people who will learn if they can see a purpose or adjust something to suit their agenda.

The challenge to you as a student is not to simply fit into this list but to roam around and experience the benefits of all styles where possible; to challenge yourself to take advantage of each style as and when needed.

 Go to the companion website to see Rosie's learning log.

Scenario 3: Supporting Development and Action Planning

This is the last week of her placement, and Blossom has been asked by her supervisor to take charge in her bay as one of her learning outcomes is related to leadership and managing care priorities on a shift. During the ward round she is asked to provide information about a woman who is having bloods sent to the lab for investigations every day. She reports the blood results to the multidisciplinary team on the round, reading from the laboratory report. One of the doctors asks Blossom to verify that the results are the most recent. Blossom looks annoyed, checks, and says, 'oh this is for 15 March' (today is 20 March). The doctor checks her electronic device and finds the most recent results for bloods taken yesterday. She reads them out. After the round, the doctor speaks to Blossom with her supervisor. 'I know it's sometimes difficult with a large group of people in front of you, but it is important that you focus and give the most up to date, accurate information. If we had not checked, we could have made wrong decisions about care.' Blossom replies 'It's your job to check the results as well, not just mine.'

Things to Think About

- What would you do?
- What are your worries?
- What are the implications of Blossom's actions?
- What might be the impact on the other students?
- What kind of conversation will you have with Blossom?

Applying Theory to Practice

This is an opportunity to support the student to understand how to take learning from an error and to develop leadership thinking.

Sometimes it is important to realise as both a supervisor and student that the student may have crossed a line in terms of adhering to safe working practice. The NMC (2018: 4.4) requires supervisors to be able 'to appropriately raise and respond to student conduct and competence concerns'.

As a supervisor you need to be able to change your leadership style from that of coach to one of directing. Situational leadership offers an excellent reminder that depending on the situation you find yourself in, you need to adopt the most relevant style.

The supervisor, discovering the error Blossom has made, needs to have more of a directing and telling conversation, leading then to coaching – rather than starting from coaching.

Exemplar of a Directing and Telling Conversation

Signposting the theory and framework of different coaching conversations.

Signposting the theory	Coaching dialogue
Assertive – establishing a directive tone.	**Supervisor:** *Blossom we need to discuss what happened today with the blood result.*
Avoidance.	**Blossom:** *It's OK thanks, it's been sorted.*
Drawing Blossom back to the seriousness of the situation.	**Supervisor:** *Blossom, you were taking charge of the bay this morning, so you are responsible for ensuring that you check and give accurate information. As a qualified midwife, you would be accountable if wrong decisions were made as a result of your error.*
Blossom is not taking accountability – hitting back at the supervisor doesn't reflect a positive working relationship of openness or trust.	**Blossom:** *How ridiculous! Anyone can make this sort of mistake! The doctors should have checked it and not relied on me.*
Open and powerful questioning.	**Supervisor:** *What could have happened as a result from your mistake and lack of checking results properly?*
Further evidence of not taking responsibility.	**Blossom:** *Well someone else would have checked instead, like in this situation.*
The seriousness of the situation is clearly communicated.	**Supervisor:** *What worries me most Blossom is your denial of the consequences of this very serious situation. Your lack of checking could have resulted in medication being given or withheld. This has important implications for the health of the woman here.*
Defensive and in denial – no real evidence of learning.	**Blossom:** *Whatever! You are being over dramatic and now victimising me! I am only a student you know! I am supposed to be supervised properly by you!*
Summary given and seriousness communicated. Working on an action plan is crucial now before any other progression can be made by Blossom.	**Supervisor:** *What has happened today requires us to work closely together to ensure that you are meeting the requirements for registration as a midwife. You should understand the accountability of a midwife and accuracy of recordkeeping is an important part of that. Communication with other professionals is a fundamental part of safe and effective care. Let's both go away and reflect on today's incident, consider what best practice would be, and make an action plan. We can all learn from every experience. Let's meet tomorrow to discuss a plan.*

Self-Learning

This offers an opportunity for you to reflect on your current practice position and what more you could do to become an even more powerful coach.

It is crucial to clearly communicate the expectations you have of students so that they know what they have to achieve. It is in this directive zone of situational leadership that there is a need to tell individuals what is expected of them and to check their understanding. Sometimes when there is evidence, as in this example, that they are not following expectations, further research is needed to find out the reasons. What is preventing Blossom from double-checking? Is it a capability issue or something to do with her attitude? What development will it take for Blossom to operate safely going forward? As a supervisor you may want to seek support to address some of these issues from either the university link lecturer or from the practice educator. Concerns about competence and action plans should be documented as part of the assessment process and communicated to the practice assessor.

The opportunity to reflect after the event provides time to examine the situation and explore the learning opportunities. The action planning exercise should help to focus on best practice for multi-professional working.

References

Nursing and Midwifery Council (2018). Standards for student supervision and assessment. https://www.nmc.org.uk/standards-for-education-and-training/standards-for-student-supervision-and-assessment (accessed 2 December 2020).

Wildflower, L. and Brennan, D. (2011). *The Handbook of Knowledge-Based Coaching: From Theory to Practice*. San Francisco: Jossey-Bass.

12

Mental Health

Rachel Paul, Charlene Lobo, Ronald Simpson and Helen Bell

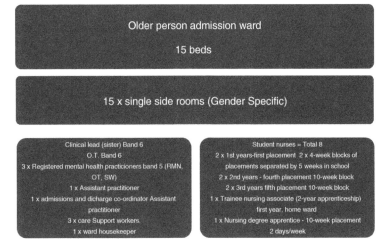

This clinical area is a 15-bedded acute admissions unit for people over the age of 65 years experiencing serious functional mental health issues, such as bipolar disorder, depression, and psychosis. It is based in a city in a rural county and it manages people with the presenting problems within a 50-mile radius.

The ward is staffed as follows: one registered nurse (RN) in charge, two other RNs and three healthcare assistants (HCA) per 7.5-hour early and late shift to care for 15 patients on the ward. In addition, there is a ward manager who works Monday to Sunday and works clinically during these times. Staffing is reduced to four on a night shift. The staff work

Collaborative Learning in Practice: Coaching to Support Student Learners in Healthcare, First Edition. Charlene Lobo, Rachel Paul, and Kenda Crozier.
© 2021 John Wiley & Sons Ltd. Published 2021 by John Wiley & Sons Ltd.
Companion website: www.wiley.com/go/lobo/collaborativelearninginpractice

as one team that each look after the ward patients. There is a full team as well as nursing staff of one consultant psychiatrist, one clinical assistant/specialist psychiatric registrar, one core trainee doctor, one foundation year-1 medical student, one clinical psychologist, one occupational therapist (Band 6), one physiotherapist, a site physical health nurse (RN adult), and a site-based clinical educator.

A clinical practice educator, Hayley, supports student nurses (direct entry and Nursing Degree Apprentices [NDAs]), new members of staff and other learners, e.g. return to practice, HCAs, and trainee nursing associates (TNAs) and is the 'nominated person' for the ward (SSSA NMC 2018). The clinical educator is dedicated to the site but works in partnership with the practice education and development team that supports clinical areas across the hospital. Hayley is an experienced clinical educator, having four years of experience in the role, and has facilitated and supported the development of four clinical wards that have adopted a contemporary collaborative model of learning. Hayley, who is the ward's education lead for learners, has worked with the ward sisters to plan the students off- duty including a rotation of multidisciplinary spoke placements to other areas such as: dementia acute admissions wards, dementia intensive support team, electroconvulsive therapy theatres and recovery, physiotherapy, occupational therapy, physical health nurse, adult acute psychiatric admissions ward, infection control team, admissions and discharge team, pharmacy, podiatry service, and the modern matron team. Students and staff usually work 8-hour days (07.00–1500 or 13.00–21.00) and 11-hour night shifts (20.30–07.30).

Students work in the same team as their practice supervisor but not necessarily their practice assessor. The clinical practice educator works on the clinical area giving both individual and group support/education to students and supervisors and supports assessors in the assessment pathway for the individual learner in the clinical environment. She identifies and addresses any clinical learning and ensures the facilitation of this. She is the link to the university assigned link lecturer and attempts to support at a level before the university needs to become involved in any issues.

Learning for students is facilitated by the practice clinical educator on the ward or by taking them to a specific clinical area to teach and let them experience clinical procedures. They also provide teaching sessions for one hour on a Wednesday and Thursday each week where a clinical specialist in a particular topic will come in and teach on that subject or use a particular clinical case study to explore and learn from.

This case study is based on the experiences of two student nurses, both of whom had six- week placements on the ward but at different times.

Scenario 1: Managing a Disgruntled Student

Alf, a third-year student, was previously an occupational therapist in another part of Europe and decided to change career to become a mental health nurse. During his preliminary interview with his practice assessor and one of his practice supervisors, he outlined his learning outcomes and how he wished to achieve these by a combination of real-time practice and supporting theory using his hub (ward) and spoke placements (see hub and spoke model in Chapter 2). He appeared to his assessors as a high-achieving student as he stated he had a degree in a health-related science. As his placement progressed, he identified his own learning needs and put himself forward for skills development, regularly jumping in before other students had the opportunity to learn. He did not volunteer to support the learning of his more junior student colleagues, although he had identified this as a learning outcome. His portfolio had not been shown to any staff members despite repeated requests in the run up to the progress meeting.

Alf requested a delay to the mid-point meeting because he had arranged a spoke placement followed by two weeks' vacation time. Unfortunately, due to clinical issues this had to be cancelled and Alf was very disappointed. He was overheard to say that he believed the ward had cancelled the spoke visit so that they could conduct the mid-point progress interview.

This scenario is based on the mid-point interview between Alf and his practice assessor (PA).

Things to Think About

- Making a split second judgement is sometimes all you can do in responding to highly charged emotions.
- Reflect on what skills you need to communicate empathy and respect for your colleagues.
- Where will you find support to discuss your responses?

Applying Theory to Practice

- The use of GROW as a model of coaching lends itself to examining behaviours required. It does not always take into account feelings, so extra work needs to happen to build and maintain rapport.
- Ego states can often be a problem in difficult conversations, making sure you keep away from parental and child ego states may help in maintain neutral but effective ways of managing difficult conversations (Harris, 1969).

 ## Exemplar of a Coaching Conversation

Signposting the theory	Coaching dialogue
Important to build rapport.	**PA:** *How are you feeling Alf?*
Feels defensive.	**Alf:** *Is something wrong?*
Clarity in **goal** of the meeting.	**PA:** *The purpose of our meeting today is to complete the mid-point a progression interview.*
Procrastination is often the result of fear.	**Alf:** *OK; although I'm not sure if I'm ready.*
Repetition of agreed reality.	**PA:** *You have had notice of this meeting for two weeks.*
Further procrastination reflecting Alf's fear,	**Alf:** *Yes, but I haven't really had much time to prepare for it.*
Evidence of email presented containing outline of outcomes expecting for assessment.	**PA:** *In this email dated two weeks ago I outlined the written work I was expecting you to provide at this meeting.*
	Alf: *What if I haven't done it yet?*
Options outlined.	**PA:** *Well, you know the process Alf; let's talk you through the assessment of practice process?*
	I am obliged to record the non-completion of these learning outcomes as a fail at this formative stage. At this point you have two options as I see it.

Signposting the theory	Coaching dialogue
	First option is you complete the outstanding assessment by Friday at 4 p.m. and this will not impact on your overall outcome.
	Second option is that we contact the link lecturer and your academic assessor, and we can sit together and formulate an action plan.
Emotions running high – *child* responses evident.	**Alf:** *So you are pushing me towards a fail, you really don't understand or care about me do you?*
It's important that the supervisor remains in adult ego state – showing support for Alf choosing an option as Alf is also an adult and he has choice.	**PA:** *Of course I care what happens here Alf; but we have an agreed assessment plan and you have not kept to the agreement, so I have a duty to follow the process but will support you in the one you choose.*
Hurt child ego state isn't helping Alf.	**Alf:** *I can't believe you are so harsh?*
Maintaining focus on solution and action not on negative.	**PA***: I don't want to be harsh Alf, I want you to complete your placement successfully! That entails handing in your written work.*
Ownership of option expressed.	**Alf:** *OK, I will go for option 1.*
When is crucial to complete the model and commitment made.	**PA:** *When by?*
When is agreed.	**Alf:** *Friday as you said – by 4 p.m.*
Collaboration evident and willingness to support will help motivate Alf.	**PA:** *What do you need from me?*
Call for support.	**Alf:** *Have faith in me?*
Reassurance needed.	**PA:** *I always do Alf*
Personal responsibility taken.	**Alf:** *Thanks – I won't let you down again.*
Check in with feelings helps to make conversation more real and powerful.	**PA:** *How are you feeling now?*
Honest response but clear commitment communicated.	**Alf:** *Exhausted but will get this writing done!*

Self-Learning

Supervisor

- How would you feel using GROW to have difficult conversations with students?
- What would the difficulties be in trying to use this model?
- How do you retain adult-to-adult ego states in resolving difficult conversations?
- What might be missing in this conversation?

Student

- How would you feel about having a conversation with your supervisor if they were using GROW?
- When could you use GROW in your working day?

 Go to the companion website to see some of the issues when considering Alf's learning journey.

Scenario 2: Managing Resistance to Learning

This scenario is the follow-up meeting as agreed between Alf and his practice assessor. The practice assessor, with agreement from Alf, asked for the HEI link lecturer to be present to support the discussion. One learning outcome that Alf had not considered was that which expected him to demonstrate his support for the learning and development of others.

Things to Think About

- How do you prepare yourself for a difficult conversation?
- What are the things you can do to look at things from someone else's perspective?
- When you are feeling at your most resourceful, what do you say to yourself?
- What do you do to research latest trends in your practice?
- When you collaborate with colleagues, what do you find works best?

Applying Theory to Practice

- Maintaining a positive rapport with learners is helpful for increasing motivation that may lead to improved performance – this links to intrinsic satisfaction (Rogers 2012: p. 134).
- What style of learning do you feel most comfortable with using Honey and Mumford's 1982 questionnaire? Activist/Theorist/Pragmatist/Reflector?
- Kolb's 1984 work on reflective learning has been used widely in different sectors, how do you use it?
- Situational leadership relies on a telling style that is arguably needed for emergency situations rather than for building learning cultures?

Exemplar of a Coaching Conversation

Signposting the theory	Coaching dialogue
Positive tone set for the discussion, which will help build rapport.	**PA:** *Well done for getting the work in Alf at the agreed time!*
Difficulties of study are clear.	**Alf:** *Thanks – As I have said, it's really hard at home and fitting in this work is really difficult to manage.*
Open probing question helps to focus discussion.	**PA:** *How do feel about discussing the learning outcome on supporting the learning and development of others?*
Alf appears unaware of the gap and its importance.	**Alf:** *OK, if you think that's relevant?*
Clear justification offered.	**PA:** *Yes, I do, as it seems to be missing in your evidence?*
Alf reflects on his approach and practice.	**Alf:** *Well I'm with the junior students teaching and showing them all the time?*
Encourage Alf to think for himself about his approach.	**PA:** *What are the limitations of this approach?*
We often use how we have been taught as a model of teaching others.	**Alf:** *None – it's how I learnt.*
Getting Alf to think in broader terms.	**LL:** *What other approaches could you be using?*

Signposting the theory	Coaching dialogue
Just because the approach has always been used doesn't mean to say it's the best approach.	**Alf:** *Well I'm not sure if there is anything better than that approach – it's been around forever!*
Gentle challenge using a neutral independent thinking approach based on independent research might stimulate reflection.	**LL:** *Yes, it has, but there is some interesting current research and feedback that we all learn differently. Therefore, as facilitators of learning, we need to make sure there is learning for everyone by making sure we vary the approaches we use a use a mix of styles.*
Alf expresses surprise, but as the assessor appears neutral by referring to recent research there is a sense of sharing and collaboration rather than a 'telling' from the directing situational leadership model, which might have felt parental or judgemental.	**Alf:** *Well that's all news to me!*
Asking Alf's opinion is more likely to engage an adult-to-adult response.	**LL:** *How are you learning now Alf?*
Alf identified for himself action he felt comfortable with that would develop his knowledge base.	**Alf:** *What? Do you mean coaching?*
Positive start to the interaction with the link lecturer plus motivation from Alf to learn more to shape his knowledge and practice of supporting the development of others.	**LL:** *Bingo Alf! Let's look at the ways you can support your peers by using a coaching approach to learning.*
Clear commitment to develop himself further from Alf.	**Alf:** *OK, let's start.*

 Self-Learning

Supervisor/practice assessor/link lecturer

- How do you support your students to take ownership of their areas of their development?

- When is it possible to share ways of working and supporting others?
- What are the ways of encouraging students to take a positive look at their practice?

Student

- How do you use the role of the link lecturer?
- When you have a difference of opinion with your assessor, what do you do?
- Where do you find support as a student?
- How do you know where to get support from as a student?

 Go to the companion website to see Alf's learning log.

Scenario 3: Developing Team Support in an Unfair World

Dianne was a second-year student who informed the ward before placement started that she was not able to work ward shifts and only 09.00–17.00 hours due to health reasons and had a letter from occupational health and university to support this. This was a complex situation for the ward who requested an urgent digital meeting with the university link lecturer and clinical educator and ward manager. A plan was developed that supported the student involvement in care and the team felt they would encourage Dianne to share her learning needs with her peers so they can also support her as part of a team of learners. However, Dianne did not interact with fellow students, and after about a week the other students began to voice their discontent and felt that Dianne was getting unfair preferential treatment.

This scenario is based on a conversation between the clinical educator (CE) and the students to develop their team support.

 Things to Think About

- How do you begin to explore with a student who has specific learning needs what support they need from you?
- What are the ways in which you will create team or peer coaching opportunities?
- Think about how you will create a positive team review in terms of the language you intend to use?

Applying Theory to Practice

- Team performance review is as short or as long as the time you have available to use it.
- Constructive feedback is a process for everyone to follow including students.

 ## Exemplar of a coaching conversation

Signposting the theory	Coaching dialogue
Leading the team to create an even more effective team going forward. Setting the scene by being open and honest with the feedback and comments made.	**CE:** *Thanks for your time and for coming together today.* *I have been told by a few of you that you feel we have given preferential treatment to Dianne and I just wanted you all to understand more about working together as a team despite the different needs of members of your team.*
Students feel free to own the feedback.	**Student 1:** *Well we just want you to understand how unfairly we feel treated. In fact, as a team we are feeling demoralised and hurt!*
Students thanked for the feedback encouraging an adult ego state. Using the meeting as an opportunity to review expectations and performance as a team.	**CE:** *OK, thank you for your honesty and openness. Let's do a bit of a review about what sort of a team we are and what we want to be?*
Seizing the moment – rather than letting negative emotions fester and grow.	**Student 2:** *What, now?*
Taking advantage of a positive learning opportunity.	**CE:** *Yes now! We need to make use of the learning created by this situation.*
Always good to have some sources of energy to help increase participation and create a team working situation.	**Student 1:** *OK, fair enough, anyone want biscuits to go with their tea? (Biscuits shared.)*

Signposting the theory	Coaching dialogue
Big opening question directed at each of the four members of the team – everyone is encouraged to participate in thinking about what makes a successful team. Give us a factor, a reason, and a rating out of 10?	**CE:** *Each of you please tell me about what you feel are the critical success factors of this team? And how important they are to you on a scale of 1 to 10.*
Each team member identified a success factor and tells the team the reason for this factor.	**Student 2:** *Honesty: we need to trust each other in order to do the right thing for the patient and each other – 8.*
The treatment of each other equally brings a smile to this student's face.	**Student 1:** *Equality: we need to treat each other the same and be treated the same – 3.*
Raised the issue indirectly of the possible reasons that Dianne had been treated differently.	**CE:** *What is equality?*
	Student 1: *We should all get the same opportunity to learn*
	CE: *What about if someone had more of a disadvantage to learning than others?*
The issue of confidentiality is key.	**Student 1:** *If we knew something like that about a team member then we would of course accept that. But no one has said anything.*
Confirmation that there are things that cannot be shared.	**CE:** *We are not able to disclose personal information about anyone. What is your factor Student 4?*
Clear reflection and making explicit the values of the team members. Kindness to self could be argued is essential for the development of professional nursing practice.	**Student 4:** *Kindness: we need to be sensitive to the needs of our patients, our doctors, each other, and ourselves. I would rate ourselves lower than the rest say at a 3?*
Keeping neutral and adult will encourage a sense of collaboration.	**CE:** *Interesting observation, thank you. Student 3?*
Great reflection on and evaluation of the role of support in the team and support for the patient.	**Student 3:** *Support: we need to be supportive of the patient's recovery in any way we are able to, support each other at times of difficulty, and support the doctors to do their jobs. I would rate this at an 8!*

Signposting the theory	Coaching dialogue
Reflective listening with ratings used to add some critical analysis.	**CE:** *OK, well done all of you; so if I can summarise then, we have honesty and support ratings at 8 but equality and kindness at 3?*
Confirmation checked and agreed.	**Student 1:** *Yes that's about it!*
Encouraging ownership of everyone to improve team performance.	**CE:** *So, as a team, let's reflect on what is needed to improve our equality and kindness in this team? Perhaps individually jot down some ideas as to what you think might be done?*
Honest and brave Student 4 has a sense of how feedback can build confidence if it is constructive. If Student 4 is feeling more confident then everyone benefits!	**Student 4:** *Let's give each other more constructive feedback? That would help my confidence and if I felt more confident about myself I might be kinder to the rest of you!*
Positively encourages the action and is specific about the timing to ensure that things will happen.	**CE:** *Sounds a good idea! When will this start and who is up for this action? I am happy to receive feedback on this team review.*
Good example of constructive feedback as well as progress made on respecting difference in the team and the different needs of the team.	**Student 4:** *Now! As a CE you are really supportive and you magically appear at the right time when we need you!* *On the other hand, we don't know a reason for why Dianne gets special treatment, but I guess as we have said that equality and kindness need to be improved I am willing to cut her some slack.*
Commitment to action from everyone and a good chance to follow up individual ratings in one-to-one catch-ups.	**CE:** *Thank you so much for this feedback and I would be interested to discuss ways in which we can all cut Dianne some slack whilst remaining realistic to the expected outcomes needed.*

 ## *Self-Learning*

Clinical Educator

- How could you encourage teams to look at how they come across as a team?
- What skills and qualities will you need to facilitate team reviews?
- When is it useful to carry out these team reviews and what else might support you?

Student

- When have you felt that someone in your team was getting special treatment and how did that make you feel?
- What action have you taken to make sure your individual needs were met as a student?

Scenario 4: Who Cares for the Supervisors?

After two weeks in practice where Dianne had been consistently intermittent in her attendance and often failed to undertake and follow through caring for patients, she decided to leave the course. The supervisors who had supported Dianne were very upset and felt their hard work to support her was not appreciated. This scenario is a conversation between the supervisors and the clinical educator.

 Things to Think About

- How do you make sure you are in a good place to manage your own feelings as a supervisor?
- When have been you able to motivate others to help access their inner resources?
- What is a positive thing you can say to yourself to help you stay calm and professional?
- When do you hold review meetings?

 Applying Theory to Practice

- Neuro-linguistic programming (NLP) is a way in which we can access greater internal resources (Ready and Burton 2004).

- Analysis of Thoughts, Feelings, and Actions as covered in Chapter 5 relate in part to cognitive approaches as well as NLP.
- Reflective practice and the work of Kolb (1984).
- Transactional analysis (TA) (Berne 1964) gives us ways of understanding ourselves internally and interpersonally by providing us with frameworks, such as the drama and winners triangle.

 ## *Exemplar of a Coaching Conversation*

Signposting the theory	Coaching dialogue
Solutions-focused opening to encourage everyone to adopt a positive mindset.	**Clinical Educator (CE):** *Thanks for your time today. I understand that you have heard the news that Dianne has left and I just want to offer you a chance to look forward and take note of any learning you may have.*
Emotions spilling out	**Supervisor 1:** *Personally, I feel really upset as we have all made such an effort with D and all her colleagues did too!*
Generalisations and negativity adding to negative 'group think'.	**Supervisor 2:** *I feel really upset too! All the extra work with reorganising timings and scheduling – it was so much work and no one appreciated that!*
Challenge using the drama triangle.	**CE:** *There is the potential to go into rescuer mode with our job and we really have to guard against that.*
Defensive but inquiring response.	**Supervisor 2:** *What do you mean by that?*
Referral to the drama triangle commonly used these days.	**CE:** *Have you heard of the drama triangle?*
Evidence of knowledge.	**Supervisor 1:** *Ah yes – Persecutor, Victim, Rescuer?*
Recognition and counter challenge with more positive 'winners triangle'.	**CE:** *Well done – yes.* *But there is also a winner's triangle, which I find a more helpful way of thinking and monitoring myself.*

Signposting the theory	Coaching dialogue
	Instead of a Persecutor we can look at this role as being proactive in giving feedback and being positive to others, recognising that most people are trying to do the best they can?
More negativity and defensiveness presented.	**Supervisor 2:** *Well I feel I have tried to do the best I could with Dianne!*
Positive actions identified.	**Supervisor 1:** *I think we both encouraged her and gave her positive feedback.*
Positive feedback offered.	**CE:** *Excellent – well done* *What did Dianne feel?*
Greater insight into how D had confided in supervisor and that it was an internal source of dissatisfaction she had identified.	**Supervisor 2:** *Dianne told me she felt out of her depth and that she kept letting everyone down.*
Open question to find out more data.	**CE:** *What was the evidence she was using to come to this conclusion?*
Indicator that D felt a victim.	**Supervisor 1:** *She didn't say – that was part of the problem, she didn't feel confident to tell us what she needed or how she felt!*
Acknowledgement of the supervisor's feelings is powerful in building positive solutions-focused outcomes.	**CE:** *That sounds frustrating for all of you?*
Pressure from the other students will have added to D's negativity of self-perception.	**Supervisor 1:** *Yes, it was, plus for the other students who felt D was getting away with an easier load due to a different schedule.*
This may have some validity as supervisors can be seen to be parental?	**Supervisor 2:** *Perhaps we did too much for her?*
Reflective listening for feelings expressed.	**CE:** *It sounds to me as though you feel it was all your responsibility?*

Signposting the theory	Coaching dialogue
Clear evidence of the rescuer and potentially a negative role without barriers and boundaries.	**Supervisor 1:** *Yes, I suppose we do!*
Reflecting on the dangers and communication of realistic expectations moving forward.	**CE:** *In order to avoid being a rescuer you have to draw up some boundaries – some parameters as to what is and isn't reasonable. We are only human beings trying to do the best we can. We outline our responsibilities to the students in their induction and then we deliver on those responsibilities. We cannot be expected to do more than that.*
Remember: change only happens in small steps – there is rarely transformational change.	**Supervisor 2:** *I get that, but I still feel guilty we couldn't do more for Dianne.*
Benefits of insight gained from the use of the model as a challenge to how realistic the expectations we have of ourselves are.	**Supervisor 1:** *It's good to be reminded of our boundaries as I know I have that rescuer potential and often feel guilty I never have enough time to support students the way I would like to!*
Linking the winner's triangle to Thoughts, Feelings, Action model used both in cognitive behaviour coaching as well as NLP (see Chapter 5).	**CE:** *Good self-awareness!* *Remember, to stop being a victim you need to voice your needs and feelings – in other words be more assertive.* *Given that awareness, what could you say to yourself that might be more helpful going forward?*
Positive reframing of a helpful thought that strengthens the resourcefulness of the supervisor going forward.	**Supervisor 1:** *I will continue to do the best I can but be clear about my boundaries, be positive towards others and assertive to avoid being a victim.*
Thoughts, Feeling, Action combined with being realistic about change.	**Supervisor 2:** *It's hard to follow that, but for me it's about having more check-in opportunities with students and focus on encouraging them to express their feelings, not leaving them bottled up resulting in negative outcomes such as leaving. Perhaps it's also the knowledge I already have which is that you cannot change anyone but you can change your response to them.*

Signposting the theory	Coaching dialogue
Further evidence of collaboration and support to encourage action.	**CE:** *What do you need from me?*
Follow up is often a great support!	**Supervisor 1:** *Review our progress supportively!*
Being held to account for what we agreed to do is helpful.	**Supervisor 2:** *Remind us of this conversation?*
Really helpful to get the action written down to encourage review of learning.	**CE:** *Don't worry, I have written this down – I will email you a copy – let's review in a month?* *What is your learning?*
Positive learning out of negative situation.	**Supervisor 1:** *That the issue of Dianne has provided us with a timely look at our expectations and role in supporting students and keeping ourselves sane!*
Key learning and greater ownership of our responsibility for what we do going forward.	**Supervisor 2:** *The same, but in addition we all have a choice in how we think, feel, and behave providing we are self-checking.*

 ## Self-Learning

- How do you facilitate a review of difficult situations?
- When and where do you communicate the expectations of roles as supervisors, students, and clinical educators?
- How are these expectations reviewed?
- What have you learned from reading this example of a conversation?
- How can you make use of this learning?

References

Berne, E. (1964). *Games People Play: The Psychology of Human Relationships*. London: Penguin.

Harris, T. (1969). *I'm Ok you're Ok: A Practical Guide to Transactional Analysis*. New York: Harper & Row.

Honey, P. and Mumford, A. (1982). *Manual of Learning Styles*. London: Peter Honey.

Kolb, D. (1984). *Experiential Learning: Experience as the Source of Learning and Development*. Upper Saddle River, NJ: Prentice Hall.

Nursing and Midwifery Council (2018) *Standards for student supervision and assessment*. www.nmc.org.uk/standards-for-education-and-training/standards-for-student-supervision-and-assessment

Ready, R. and Burton, K. (2004). *Neuro-Linguistic Programming for Dummies*. Chichester: Wiley.

Rogers, J. (2012). *Coaching Skills – A Handbook*, 3e. Maidenhead: McGraw-Hill.

Conclusion

Kenda Crozier, David Huggins, Charlene Lobo and Rachel Paul

Throughout this book we have examined ways to improve the learning experience of students in practice settings to enable them to be prepared for their role as qualified practitioners at the end of their programmes. We have provided a model that adopts a systems wide approach to practice education and is based on collaborative partnership between education and health service providers. The examples of coaching theories and models and coaching conversations demonstrate how learning can be supported. But fundamental to this is that learners and their practice educators need to find the opportunities for learning in busy clinical environments (Sholl et al. 2017). Whilst educators juggle their clinical workload and student supervision so that patient safety and patient outcomes are positively impacted by the learning environment, the impetus must be on the higher organisational management to ensure that learning is a recognised and valued culture. Investment has been identified by many authors as important to achieving high-quality learning environments, so before concluding we want to offer up a cautionary tale.

The Importance of Sustainable Systems of Student Support

Here we present a composite picture of a number of issues that have arisen across sites, that is provided to enable those supporting coaching

Collaborative Learning in Practice: Coaching to Support Student Learners in Healthcare,
First Edition. Charlene Lobo, Rachel Paul, and Kenda Crozier.
© 2021 John Wiley & Sons Ltd. Published 2021 by John Wiley & Sons Ltd.
Companion website: www.wiley.com/go/lobo/collaborativelearninginpractice

models to be vigilant to mission drift, which has potential to undermine the effectiveness of the learning environment. In this composite we have a fictionalised practice environment which we have called Canary ward to provide illustration.

Canary ward is regarded as a 'flagship' coaching area for the organisation, being an early adopter of CLiP™. Before implementing coaching, an educational audit was performed to identify how many students could be supported within the learning environment using the CLiP model. This model enabled learner numbers to increase from 6 before implementation to 14 during the CLiP pilot. Investment was provided for a clinical educator (CE) who provided coaching training, support, and guidance to staff, as well as ensuring that the model was implemented as envisaged and agreed. At the end of the pilot project, students and staff indicated that Canary ward was exemplifying the key principles, including identifying learning outcomes, using effective coaching conversations (Clutterbuck and Megginson 2006), using the CLiP learning hour, student presentations, and learning logs to demonstrate a high-value, quality learning experience.

In the years since the pilot project ended, Canary ward has experienced some organisational changes which have impacted on coaching effectiveness. The ward is experiencing challenges associated with the coaching approach being less evident and a more traditional model of supporting learners reappearing. This case study aims to demonstrate how mission drift (Cornforth 2014) can occur and will look at what can be done to support key coaching principles during times of organisational and educational change and support practice areas in preventing drift.

Increasing Student Numbers

CLiP was regarded as successful in increasing placement capacity for learners and reducing the 'burden' of mentorship on staff (Carlisle et al. 2009; Lascelles 2010; Wisdom 2011; Lobo et al. 2014). The model encouraged all staff working to support learning and assessment by participating in a coaching approach, and this is what enabled larger numbers than traditional placement approaches. Canary ward has seen further growth in learner numbers in response to increased recruitment required for future workforce planning, and now supports up to 22 students at a time. Whilst the increase in numbers is agreed through an audit process, this is based on the assumption that the CLiP model is in place. Other associated factors with potential to negatively impact are:

1. Variation in programmes being supported by the practice area – includes three year traditional nursing degree, two year masters, nursing degree apprenticeships, nursing associate programmes.
2. Different programmes articulating learning outcomes in different ways.
3. Practice assessment documents varying according to programme or educational institution.
4. Lack of preparation in coaching principles for students and new staff.
5. New NMC standards for education which have introduced new terminology and processes (practice supervisors, practice assessors, academic assessors).
6. Different approaches to protected learning time and supernumerary status.

Whilst changes have been communicated, there may have been challenges in reaching all staff at the right time. Staff have been recruited from outside the area so that many are not familiar with CLiP and coaching principles. Whilst a coaching approach should be used for all learners, many staff have become concerned about the new learner roles and what they can or cannot do in practice. Staff feel frustrated and unsure of learning outcomes that need to be met and they struggle to have the time to undertake supervision and assessment of students effectively. Due to diminishing numbers of experienced coaches, there is a risk that the coaching approach could be lost from practice. These difficulties are compounded by organisational change which has seen support from clinical educators altered as their numbers have reduced.

The learner experience has also suffered, with students sensing the unease of staff, now reporting that they are used as a pair of hands rather than learning and on occasions unable to achieve some of the learning outcomes. The impact of reduction in use of the CLiP learning hour alongside the lack of clinical educator time means that the ethos of a clinical learning environment is under threat.

Preparation for Coaching

Coaching training consisted of a three-tier approach for staff and a single coaching preparation session for students, which was timetabled as part of preparation for practice. Training was also provided for relevant academic staff who would be supporting the first wave of coaching wards/departments with staff attending either session 1 or 2 provided for trust staff.

The three-tier training for staff consisted of level 1 coaching training that focused on CLiP and basic coaching elements. A coaching day was discussed along with relevant processes such as learning logs, the CLiP learning hour, and student presentations. All staff were expected to participate in coaching of students and we now see this ethos being applied in the NMC standards (NMC 2018). Level 1 training was held at the university and also delivered within the trust; Level 2 recapped on Level 1 key issues but then focused on coaching models such as GROW (Whitmore 2009) and specific skills associated with coaching students, such as utilising a questioning approach and coaching conversations to enable students to identify their own learning needs. Level 2 training was targeted at experienced mentors (NMC 2008) and academic staff, although ward staff could attend if available.

Level 3 training was a two-day programme focused on developing clinical educators to support coaching in practice and to prepare them for this role. Day 1 consisted of in-depth training and support in coaching models and educational theory and Day 2 was aimed at developing leadership and management skills for their new role.

Since the end of the project, coaching training both within university and the ward has reduced significantly. Students still get an introduction to coaching in the 'preparation for placements' session and during trust induction days. Significantly, new staff commencing on the ward may be unfamiliar with the coaching model and therefore the capacity for coaching has diminished within the staff group. Experienced senior staff who were fundamental in supporting and driving a coaching approach to learning have left the ward. Clinical educator roles in supporting wards have also changed focus. In short, this means that many newer and existing coaching areas are still fundamentally not clear on the principles of coaching that are promoted within the trust. These are issues which are beyond the control of one ward or practice area and these organisational issues need to be addressed through educational partnership collaborations.

Students are also less well prepared and often face a busy work area where they are allocated to a coaching ward, explained the principles and processes to expect, but find these are not carried out. There is also limited support to seek further guidance and advice when on placement.

Clinical Educator and Link Lecturer Support

A role that was identified as pivotal in supporting coaching training and development was that of the clinical educator (Hill et al. 2015). Within the original CLiP project, designated CEs were trained and educated in promoting coaching. CEs attended all tiers of coaching training and worked alongside academic staff when delivering training sessions to trust-based staff in the clinical area. This ensured a consistent approach to all coaching placement areas. Since the end of the pilot project, training and updating of existing and new educators has altered to providing updates on NMC standards and the online practice assessment document in a generic way. Often staff undertaking this role are new to a senior education role and lack confidence in the model and have limited knowledge of coaching – and thus are not able to make the clear links between the coaching approach and the NMC standards. Training for university staff in link lecturer roles has seen similar issues arise. Practice development teams have recognised the need to develop training in supporting the role of clinical educators and are finding ways in which career development opportunities for progression to these roles can be supported by education.

New NMC Standards

Throughout every clinical placement, relevant professional body standards overarch the support of learners in practice. The original CLiP project needed to take account of the NMC Supporting Learning and Assessment in Practice (2008) standards. In 2018, the NMC introduced new education standards, which included Standards to Support Student Supervision and Assessment in Practice (SSSA) (NMC 2018). These new standards are well suited to the coaching model. The practice supervisor role fits with the role of coach, the practice assessor role and the academic assessor role are all contained within the CLiP model.

As staff are trying to learn the new processes, concentration on the existing skills of coaching may have slipped. An opportunity may have been lost by not linking the role of the practice supervisor to that of coach. Indeed, there is evidence that the role of a coaching supervisor has benefits for one-to-one learning. Bodies such as the International Coaching Federation (ICF) see coaching supervision as a process of 'collaborative learning practice' that continually builds the capacity of the coach through reflective dialogue for the benefit of both coaches and clients (in this case learners). The advantages of coaching supervision, such as increased self-awareness, greater confidence, increase objectivity, and a heightened sense of belonging, were recognised by Tkach and DiGirolamo (2017) as key benefits for people receiving coaching supervision. It could be argued that with the popularity of coaching strategies being used heavily in healthcare learning, the linking of coaching and supervision could have been thought through in a little more detail. The change from mentor/coach to supervisor and assessor has ultimately been seen by staff as simply being a number of completely new changes to supporting learning in clinical practice rather than something to be carried forward and utilised correctly to support the new standards. This may be due to the university staff overlooking the need to make the links explicit.

Partly Applying the Model

A fundamental aspect of introducing a coaching philosophy to clinical practice was ensuring that there was a clear theoretical underpinning – albeit a stronger leaning towards coaching theories rather than pure education theory. CLiP introduced standard resources to cover subjects such as the 'ideal' coaching day, establishing learning outcomes, time out (CLiP hour) for students to spend time research learning on shift, and criteria for student presentations. The use of the framework for facilitating learning (based on the situational model) ensured students were allocated to patient care commensurate with their competence and abilities and not on the basis of their year group. Students were advised on their role in coaching other students. However, during the project, it was clear that individual areas were adapting the coaching approach to suit local need and a certain degree of 'coaching hybridisation' was occurring. This leads to confusion when students or staff move within an organisation and find different approaches being taken.

Lessons Learned

Collaborative educational partnerships – the setting up of the CLiP project had seen excellent collaboration in developing working practice, supporting students and staff, as well as developing networks. Whilst there is still collaborative working in place, the level of intensity of this in supporting the growth of a coaching organisation has lessened – especially at the organisational level. This is further complicated as the numbers of educational partners grow. The collaboration on approaches to supporting students must extend across all partners for true collaboration and shared vision to be enacted. Leadership within the practice organisation is required to insist that all practitioners apply the same principles of coaching to ensure a consistent approach within the learning environment. High-quality practice education requires constant review of processes and standards to ensure maintenance.

Need for consistent communication of key messages – It can be seen that a unified approach between all parties around the fundamental parameters of how a coaching approach is to support learning is beneficial to all parties participating in the process. This will minimise the dilution and adaptation of key coaching components, models, and theories within each different organisation, leading to parity of coaching practices in the clinical area.

Training of new staff – there needs to be a unified, standardised approach to preparing staff and students in key coaching principles for implementation into the clinical learning environment. The responsibility for quality in practice learning should be agreed between partners so that educational updates remain part of the culture. The success of the CLiP project indicated that this was a key element in the success of coaching. A vital aspect of this is ensuring that clinical educators are fully trained in coaching and education theory to be a consistent source of support for staff and students in practice. Specific training involving relevant partners, such as universities, that looks not just to coaching but to the overall role and responsibilities of clinical educators could be developed with emphasis on coaching principles being at the forefront.

Need for education leadership role in times of change – organisations are in a constant state of flux in response to changes in healthcare policy, but it is important that an educational perspective is kept in plain view at the top of organisations. This should involve and inform directors of nursing, members of hospital boards, professional leads, and deans of health schools. This partnership in leadership is pivotal in ensuring consistent messages of the benefits of coaching throughout the complex layers of a learning organisation.

Coaching leadership – coaching leadership is seen by Robertson (2016) as a process developed around building leadership capacity in individuals, and in institutions, through enhancing professional relationships. It is based on the importance of maximising potential, and harnessing the ongoing commitment and energy needed to meet personal and professional goals. Where coaching is seen in action across all levels of organisation, it is easier to apply coaching to practice education.

Recommendations

It is inevitable that changes will occur in a learning environment as staff turnover occurs and changes take place at an organisational level that impact on care delivery. Investment is required to ensure sustainability of a coaching model particularly, as it is so well suited to the NMC standards for student support and assessment. It is important that commitment is made to maintain quality as this will ensure a workforce in the future that is also familiar with high standards in practice education and a culture of learning. Education of new staff is important, and this includes new clinical educators, which are not to be regarded as an addition but as an integral part of the clinical learning environment. Clinical educator roles require educational support and recognition by qualification, so development of programmes to support them should be a goal of partnerships between practice partners and education institutions. The role of university lecturers in support for practice learning should be clearly articulated and universities and practice organisations should review agreements to ensure that these are included. The education institutions should work collaboratively with practice to ensure that an audit of practice areas is completed in a timely way and that it focuses on ensuring learning environments are effective as well as safe. Coaching models work best within organisations that support coaching across all levels of the organisation. Further educational research is needed on support of students. It is clear from the research to date that one size does not fit all. Much research is focused on the experience of supervisors, students, clinical practice educators, and faculty. There needs to be some focus on the experience of patients and clients of health professional students and cost analysis of the models as they are developed. The sustainability of practice education models must be factored into the cost of educating health students to enable funding to be realistically established. New curricula are being developed all over the UK in response to changes in NMC standards for nursing and midwifery education and it is important that these are properly evaluated. Attention also needs to be paid to support of newly qualified staff as they develop in confidence.

References

Carlisle, C., Calman, L., and Ibbotson, T. (2009). *Practice-based learning: the role of practice education facilitators in supporting mentors. Nurse Education Today* 29 (7): 715–721.

Clutterbuck, D. and Megginson, D. (2006). *Making Coaching Work. Creating a Coaching Culture.* CIPD-Kogan Page.

Cornforth, C. (2014). *Understanding and combating mission drift in social enterprises.* Corporate governance. An international review. *Social Enterprise Journal* 7 (4): 346–362.

Hill, R., Woodward, M., and Arthur, A. (2015). *Collaborative Learning in Practice (CLiP): Evaluation Report.* East Anglia: HEE East of England and University of East Anglia.

Lascelles, M.A. (2010). Students' and mentors' experiences of mentoring and learning to practice during the first year of an accelerated programme leading to nurse registration. PhD thesis. University of Leeds.

Lobo, C., Arthur, A. and Latimmer, V. (2014). Collaborative Learning in Practice (CLiP) for pre-registration nursing students; a background paper for delegates attending the CLiP conference. University of East Anglia and NHS Health Education East of England. Norwich.

NMC (2008). *Standards to Support Learning and Assessment in Practice.* London: Nursing and Midwifery Council.

Nursing and Midwifery Council (2018). *Realising Professionalism: Standards for Education and Training. Part 2: Standards for Student Supervision and Assessment*, 2018. London: NMC.

Robertson, J. (2016). *Coaching Leadership. Building Educational Leadership Capacity through Partnerships*, 2e. Wellington NZCER Press.

Sholl, S., Ajjawi, R., Allbutt, H. et al. (2017). *Balancing health care education and patient care in the UK workplace: a realist synthesis. Medical Education* 51: 787–801.

Tkach, J.T. and DiGirolamo, J.A. (2017). The state and future of coaching supervision. *International Coaching Psychology Review* 12: 49–63.

Whitmore, J. (2009). *Coaching for Performance. GROWing Human Potential and Purpose. The Principles and Practice of Coaching Leadership*, 4e. Nicholas Brearley Publishing.

Wisdom, H. (2011). Mentors' experiences of supporting pre-registration nursing students. A grounded theory study. Thesis. The Open University.

Index

Collaborative Learning in Practice: Coaching to Support Student Learners in Healthcare,
First Edition. Charlene Lobo, Rachel Paul, and Kenda Crozier.
© 2021 John Wiley & Sons Ltd. Published 2021 by John Wiley & Sons Ltd.
Companion website: www.wiley.com/go/lobo/collaborativelearninginpractice